GIRLS! 7 REASONS WHY CALORIES IN, CALORIES OUT DON'T COUNT!

SENSATIONAL METABOLIC HEALTH AND HAPPINESS FOR LIFE!

COACH BLADE

CONTENTS

For additional tips, support, and to take an active role in your health and wellbeing, please don't hesitate to reach out!

Discover more on my website:

https://iscfitness.co.uk/

And get involved by joining our community on Facebook:

https://www.facebook.com/ISCFitnessUK/

I'll see you there!

INTRODUCTION

Hello, Girls! Before we get this journey together started, I feel it is only proper to introduce myself and let you know the reasons why you should be taking any notice of what I'm telling you.

Let us start with a little bit about me as a business. I created the brand ISCF (Ian Stanley Community Fitness) around five years ago to link all the aspects of my health and fitness business under one fab umbrella. At the start of my career, I was a personal trainer, primarily focused on one to one training. After that, I started teaching and coaching classes inside the gyms, which progressed to teaching special needs sessions over time. As my career began to gather momentum and my schedule became swamped, I added the fantastic dimension of Olympic Lifting and functional training to further increase my service's quality (which I still use today).

Today, I work almost exclusively online. After being inside gyms for the best part of 20+ years, I felt it was time to evolve and take my business to the next level. I am now coaching clients from all over the UK and overseas. I have some sessions outside for the hardcore, especially given the typical British weather. Which brings me to this book... Becoming a published author was the one media format I had not explored, and it seemed like an excellent way to get my message out to the world!

So, as you can clearly see, girls, I have had so many years developing my skills and perfecting my craft to become the best coach and trainer I can be. Most of my clients over the years have been girls. Even when I opened my own CrossFit Box in 2012, we attracted warrior ladies from all over the area who wanted to learn from Coach Blade! Oh! and I think I better just let you know at this point that the nickname Blade came from so long ago now I cannot even remember its origins, but it's stuck! And everyone knows me by that name, so I humbly accept it and use it with pride!

But we're getting ahead of ourselves. As I was saying, I've worked with and alongside many girls, and I've become much more than just a coach and PT for them. I have become an all-around life coach and assistant, if you will, offering much more than just training. For example, I have gone shopping with clients to help them make better and wiser food choices. They tell me in detail how their bodies are reacting to certain types of foods and new training moves and, crucially, helped them get away from calorie counting!

Now, I know that you may still be skeptical at this point and may need a little more convincing. Well, not only will you find this book very informative and laid out very simply so that we can all understand the reasons, but it should be entertaining too! If there is one thing you should know about me, it's that I am not a "doom and gloom" type of guy! That said, some of the things I talk about in this book go against the grain, against the "dogma" of what the majority are telling us. And we are fully aware that many of the reasons we give as to why we don't even need to think about calories, let alone count them, go totally against the advice of almost all other diets, health books, and magazines. However, in all my 25 years in this field, counting calories always fails. For sure, in the short term, there is some weight loss, but as I'll explain in great detail later in this book, it is not from the numbers that the body loses, but the ability to speak the body's language. So, guess what??!! You are going to learn a brand new language! By the end of this book, you will understand your body more and communicate with it better!

Also, throughout this book, you will find lots of hints and tips to help our fantastic vegan and veggie warriors! Although this is not a diet book in the typical sense of the word, we will constantly be directing and coaching our readers to find a path that suits them best for optimal health. Once you discover this path for yourself, it is a BIG eureka moment!

As we've always said (and my veggie and vegan girls and boys agree with me on this too), it is not our job to tell you what you should or shouldn't be eating, especially when it comes to your beliefs. If you do not want to eat any animal products whatsoever, we will fully support that choice. However, it *is* our job to help you become fitter, stronger, and healthier ladies! For instance, if you enjoy a diet of all plants and no animal products, you will miss many essential vitamins and minerals, so you have to be careful to compensate. We will cover these in more detail later in the book. So, don't worry, we got you! As your coach, I must advise taking supplements that fill the void left by the lack of meats and animal products. You can and will live a fab and on-fire life without certain products or produce, but we need to fill the blanks in. Essential vitamins, proteins, and minerals are precisely that: essential. The body needs them to thrive. Supplementation and carefully selecting the correct veggies, seeds, nuts, and oils help a great deal. We are fully supportive of all and any beliefs, and all are very welcome here. We are an optimal health and fitness setup! And as such, you will need to put the correct food in to reap the benefits, and we will help do just that.

But on a more serious note, it's vital to be aware that we are in a world of peer pressure and body image problems right now. Some even say it is a crisis. Girls of all ages are trying to "live up" to the Insta crowd! It's brutally harsh. To look a certain way! To do what others are doing! I WILL NOT stand to the side and watch this story unfold, especially when I have seen so many terrible situations with girls wanting to end it all because of the pressures and thinking that calories are the answer.

Your body will shut down if you undereat! It is trying to survive! You CANNOT bully your body into dropping its body fat and then become more healthy!

However, if you learn to talk to your body, to converse with it each day, listen to it, and feed it correctly after, then not only will you become leaner and more toned, but the health and freedom benefits come along too!

But why should you listen to me and follow the advice in this book? Well, we believe we are helping to dispel the myth around calorie counting forever! And in the process, remove the powerful "dogma" that drives millions of girls from around the world to "follow the crowd" and ultimately fail in their pursuit of low body fat and better health. We must be brave warriors because the trail we blaze is not on the path we are told to follow. But we are not sheep! The girls who are reading this book want a different way! A way that ultimately leads to freedom from counting and weighing anything ever again! You need to be able to talk to your body, feed it correctly, intuitively knowing what foods to choose and to leave out. You need to be comfortable with who you are right now and take steps to be so much better! You can have better health! Improved fitness! More energy! Better sleep! Less metabolic illness!

The list is endless! Be one of our new wave girls! Use this book and its teachings to discover ultimate freedom and a way of living life to the max!

And so, come with us. Let us begin...

Most people believe long-term weight loss is simply about cutting a few calories here and there. Sure, it sounds like it works, but the bottom line is that it does not. In fact, most dieters will tell you that they tried this and it didn't work. So, what's the problem? The problem is that most of us think about weight loss as a temporary situation. This is not how it should be. Our bodies are designed to be in a state of constant weight control, and when we routinely de-train our bodies from this process for even a few weeks (and we normally do), our metabolism will quickly reset itself to return to pre-dieting levels. Consider the following true story.

A lady, Rael, goes on vacation to Mexico for a two-week break from her normal routine. While on the trip, she decides to lose weight by dramatically reducing her calorie intake. For two weeks, she eats 30% fewer calories than is recommended for her (or so we are told by the government, despite how obesity and metabolic illnesses have all exploded worldwide). She returns from vacation two weeks later, weighing about five pounds less than she did when she started the trip. However, once back home again, Rael is quickly back to her normal routine and eating habits. Within just a few weeks of returning home, Rael has gained every pound back and then some. Her body has adjusted itself to the new weight.

Most people take their bodies back to their normal weight after the diet because our metabolism slows down over time, and as we reduce our calorie intake, it will do the same. This means that if one were to reduce her calorie intake for many weeks continuously, she would slowly lose strength in her arms, legs, and all parts of her body. Her muscles would become weaker as they used less oxygen and glucose required for energy, meaning she would need more oxygen and glucose to perform daily tasks such as walking. To achieve permanent, long-term weight loss, the key is not to count calories but to keep carbohydrates and sugars low, which keeps insulin levels low so that fat is burned as energy for the body. Interestingly, This is always the case with weight loss because we have a term called "weight set-point," which is our body's natural tendency to reach a stable equilibrium in weight.

The fact of the matter is that most people who try to lose weight through dieting find themselves back at their original weight within a few weeks. So if you want results, you need to focus on making the right changes in your life that will last for good. It may be difficult to ensure that you are losing more energy from your body when it comes to losing weight. However, there are many things that you can do to increase the amount of energy you burn to reach your weight loss goals.

By taking the necessary steps in consideration of your needs and exercise routine, weight loss will help keep up with all other changes that have been made to this point, such as eating less sugar and more vegetables and healthy foods. That is how our body's metabolism is affected. This is because every piece of food you eat has to be broken down into its smallest component, forcing the body to deal with each element very differently. These components are protein, fat, and glucose.

There are 4 main areas to look at in regard to weight loss. Firstly, A healthy lifestyle can help anyone achieve lifetime weight loss, but it does not happen overnight. The first step is to start on a good diet and exercise program. When it comes to exercise, you are probably familiar with the high-intensity workouts at the gym or your local health club. These can be very effective for losing weight and are superb for the busy lady who needs a workout but is limited on time. However, with the proper diet and adequate time, they can help you lose weight without doing them so often.

In fact, calories do not influence our fat stores. The other three are:

- Your metabolism
- Your body's water and muscle content
- Your exercise habits.

Your metabolism determines how quickly your body uses energy. Just as important is exercise since this helps you maintain a healthy and active lifestyle. The body uses energy in fat in carbohydrate form during exercise, which can help you lose weight. The goal is to burn energy and keep insulin low to allow the fat to be used as the body's primary fuel since your body needs the energy to stay healthy, but it does not store extra fuel for that purpose. Our bodies store up fat, which is then utilized as fuel when a hormonal signal is given. The body will either use the glucose we have stored or go back to the liver and create its own glucose to be used. Glucose is needed in every cell in the body for energy. However, the body is an amazing bit of kit! It will make glucose if there is a shortage. But do not panic! This is a perfectly natural system that kicks in when it is needed. We do not have to consume large quantities of refined carbs and sugar to top-up our stores. The body uses *less* energy at rest, and if we have low sugars and carbs in our belly, it results in nice low blood sugar levels. The excess sugar is converted to fat and stored as triglycerides in our fat cells. When we exercise, we burn off these fat cells and use glucose in our muscles as energy.

So, a very simple equation for you girls is:

More carbs and sugar you eat = More body fat stored

Fewer carbs and sugar you eat = Less body fat stored

And the best thing about this is you are now talking to your body! Oh Yes! You have started to learn the language and use it. Making this one move has now got your body listening!

Counting calories in and calories out are not needed when it comes to losing weight. The key lies in how low and stable we can keep our blood sugar. By simply exercising a few times a week, we can increase our body's ability to use the fat stores it takes in every day. When we eat our food, our bodies immediately burn off the available sugars and carbs first to digest our food and store the rest, either as fat or glycogen (the latter is used when exercising, and your body needs energy).

- If you reduce calorie intake, your total energy expenditure also decreases.
- If your body does not receive the required amount of nutrients, it can slow its BMI to compensate for your metabolic rate becoming weaker.
- Calorie In and Calorie Out diet plans sets forth a false belief that eating is your conscious decision and you can control it.

For a long time, we have believed that our bodies' ability to process calories is what determines whether we become obese or not. This is indicated in the equation below:

3500 calories = 1 pound of fat (Not true!)

Under eat by 500 calories a day and X that by 7 days = 3500 calories

This then means you will lose 1 pound of fat per week.

PROBLEM - It is technically impossible to balance your calories in with your calories out!

While the above equation appears to be correct, there are numerous assumptions tied to it. Let's look at some of them:

Assumption 1

Calories In and Calories Out are independent of each other.

There exists a strong relationship between the calories consumed and those expended. When a person reduces the number of calories they consume, the body also reduces how much energy it expends, which leads to marginal weight loss. So, staying with the numbers for a while to play devil's advocate, the experts and dogma tell us to believe that the reduction in calories will come from our fat stores and that the body will simply let go of these calories. Well, do we really think our body is that stupid? It wants to survive. Our DNA is programmed to keep us alive at any cost. So, as we feed it less (calorie reduction), we expect the body to continue to run all its systems at full capacity creating the "Calorie deficit." Please! That doesn't make any sense, right? As we have said, if you drop the food, the body will start to shut down to compensate. If you try harder and drop the food even more, the body will follow you by shutting down even further. It WILL NOT just continue to run on all cylinders while you feed it less!

Assumption 2

The basal metabolic rate is stable.

Our BMR (Basal Metabolic Rate) is the amount of energy our body needs each day to survive to operate all its systems perfectly over a 24-hour period. The problem here, girls, is that it has once again been given a calorie number! This also drives me crazy! Because our body is not an extensive collection of numbers! You are flesh and blood and nerves and bones, with not one number anywhere. Plus, diets and dieters say that all girls use around the same amount of calories. But how can that be? You are all beautifully different! All amazing sizes and shapes, so how can one girl's energy needs be the same as another's?

Assumption 3

We exert control over Calories In.

It is important to note that various hormonal systems influence when to eat and when to stop. We, therefore, cannot control the number of Calories In or Calories Out.

Assumption 4

Fat stores are not regulated and can be burned easily at will.

Fat stores are very well-regulated, using the insulin hormone as a trigger to store fat or burn it.

If this is true, and it is, why do we assume that the body, while only reacting to hormones and the changes to them, will suddenly start to use a number scale instead? Well, It won't!

And yet, all of the diets and health advice we are given is built around this counting theory!

Specific hormones regulate all our body systems. A hormone ABSOLUTELY regulates fat growth! It has nothing to do with the amount of food but the amount of carbs and sugar. Hormones that regulate fat growth are leptin and adiponectin. The fact that hormones regulate fat growth makes obesity a hormonal issue, not a caloric issue.

Assumption 5

All calories are the same.

We cannot reduce all foods to their caloric energy. For example, is the metabolic response of a calorie of sugar similar to that of olive oil? A calorie of sugar leads to an increase in blood sugar levels which prompts the pancreas to produce insulin. On the other hand, a calorie of olive oil does not increase blood sugar levels.

How Do We Process Food?

All the food that we consume contains three macronutrients: fat, protein, and carbohydrates. Once they enter the stomach, they mix with acids and, once digested, are gradually released into the small intestine. Nutrients are extracted along the way, and whatever remains is expelled from the body as stool.

Proteins are broken down into amino acids and then used to repair body tissues. Whatever is left over after this process is then stored. Fats are absorbed directly, while carbohydrates are broken down into sugars. The body gets all the energy it needs from fats, proteins, and carbohydrates, but each undergoes a different metabolic process.

Calorie Reduction Is Not the Primary Factor in Weight Loss

Even though there has been a rise in obesity, research has proven no relationship between an increase in calorie consumption and weight gain. The explosion in obesity and other health issues is primarily due to the consumption of highly processed foods. Large quantities of refined carbs and sugar have become a big part of everyday meals.

The biggest reason for all the processing is profit! Simple as that! The big companies are constantly trying to find new ways of extending the shelf life of their products. You see, if a product can stay on the shelf for six months or so, it has a greater chance of selling. If it goes bad too quickly, the company that makes the product may lose money. Our health IS NOT high on the priority list of company standards, I can assure you! Plus, processed goods are loaded with sugars and nasty salts, meaning that they taste delicious, which is very powerful and drives us to buy more. The dopamine receptors in the brain are hit hard by sugar which gives us that "high" rush feeling, the exact same receptors class A drugs hit! So you see, this is a very smart and calculated strategy to get us all coming back for more time and time again, making the company more money!

Now, of course, buying processed goods, while many products are bad, not all of them are, and if we are smart, certain ones can help. For example, dried fruit has a long shelf life but is relatively healthy. Also, tinned meats, while high in salt, are low in sugars, certainly, a better choice than no meat at all when used sparingly.

A little more science stuff here, girls! Sometimes, all we need are the facts, but other times, we need a little more information to discover for ourselves how our body works.

The First Law of Thermodynamics states that energy can neither be created nor destroyed in an isolated system. Our bodies are not isolated systems. There is constant energy going in and out, so the law does not apply.

If an individual consumes 2000 calories in a day, they can be used for digestion, cognition, breathing, and some are expelled from the body as stool. Interestingly, we are less concerned when the calories are used to facilitate body functions, but we have a problem when they are stored as fat.

Caloric Reduction: Extreme Experiments, Unexpected Results

The truth is, a caloric reduction leads to some weight loss initially, but in the long run, it's not an effective option. At the beginning of a caloric reduction diet, one might experience intense physical and psychological changes such as reduced heart rate, reduction in body temperature, drop in blood pressure, loss of hair, or lack of interest in anything besides food.

A reduction in caloric intake will reduce how much energy the body expends in managing bodily functions. Like I said just a moment ago, the body adapts because it does not want to die. If it doesn't, all protein and fat stores will be exhausted, and the individual will die. So, before the body shuts down, it will do what it can to reduce energy consumption for as long as it can.

Many people who have tried to eat less in their quest to lose weight seem not to be losing any weight in the long run. Caloric reduction diets do not work.

Hunger Games

The decision to use the Calories In and Calories Out concept assumes that we have the conscious ability to control what we eat as humans. When we reduce calorie intake, the body reduces energy expenditure, and hormones start sending us signals to eat to regain the lost weight. Weight loss has a significant impact on the hormone that makes us hungry: ghrelin. Hormones that make us feel full, like peptide YY, amylin, and cholecystokinin, are also affected.

The Vicious Cycle of Under-Eating

When we start eating less to lose weight, our metabolism reduces, and our hunger signals amplify. We continue to eat less, and over time we become tired, cold, and hungry, and before long, we go back to our old eating habits, and the weight comes back immediately. The cycle begins again. Even though we are only doing what our hormones are influencing us to do, we end up feeling like failures.

The Cruel Hoax

It is awful to blame yourself for your inability to lose weight and keep it off using caloric reduction. Pharmaceutical companies have also come up with pills intended to block the absorption of dietary fats. Although as we know, fat is not the enemy! We want the fat in our diet to be up to replace the horrid refined carbs and sugars. Fat WILL NOT raise blood sugar and will keep insulin low, thus allowing the body fat to be burned off. They also don't tell you that these fat-blocking pills come with numerous side effects since the unabsorbed fat comes out the other end, leading to stained underwear and potential damage to body organs like the liver. The truth of the matter is that neither the calorie reduction diet nor the pills work.

REASON ONE: DOGMA

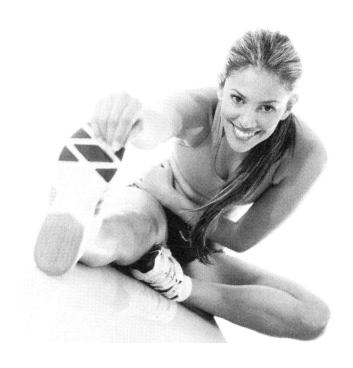

RIGHT, here we go... Below is a short story that shows "Dogma" in its powerful, insidious, and horrid form! And as you read it, put yourself in that year, in that hospital, right there! And, ask yourself this question: what if you were the one just about to have a baby? What if it was you who thought, "I hope I don't die while I give birth. I have heard such terrible things regarding new mothers."

There was a time when a doctor could work on a dead body in one room, then WITHOUT WASHING THEIR HANDS OR USING ANY FORM OF DISINFECTANT, swap rooms and help a lady give birth, and NO ONE thought anything was wrong! It would cause uproar now, right? And rightly so! When a young, smart physician suggested that if they only washed their hands between rooms, it could almost stop all mortality on the spot, he was almost laughed at!

He KNEW something was not right. He KNEW that small, microscopic "things" were being passed on to the girls in labor, and yet the large and powerful medical profession did not believe him. At that time, he couldn't prove it. The technology was not around then, so he was stripped of his license and eventually driven to madness, still working to prove his theory. But as you read this story, bring it up to date, but consider the calorie counting "dogma." Now, of course, I understand that it's not life or death as obviously as the example above, but not all problems are acute! Long-term health issues are chronic. They take time to work their evil magic. So no, of course, we won't drop dead on the spot if we count calories! But, the long-term effects can be terrible.

The "dogma" we face is the popular assumption that counting calories is the only way. It is NOT! We are fighting to forge our own path, away from this dogma!

Ignaz Philipp Semmelweis[1] is a Hungarian physician who discovered the cause of puerperal (childbed) fever and introduced antisepsis into medical practice. Educated at the universities of Pest and Vienna, Semmelweis received his doctorate from Vienna in 1844 and was appointed assistant at the obstetric clinic in Vienna. He soon became involved in the problem of puerperal infection, the scourge of maternity hospitals throughout Europe. Although most women at the time delivered at home, some sought hospitalization because of poverty, illegitimacy, or obstetrical complications. Mortality rates ranged as high as 25–30 percent. Some thought that the infection was induced by overcrowding, poor ventilation, the onset of lactation, or miasma. Semmelweis proceeded to investigate its cause over the strong objections of his chief, who, like other continental physicians, had reconciled himself to the idea that the disease was unpreventable.

Semmelweis observed that, among women in the first clinic division, the death rate from childbed fever was twice or three times as high as among those in the second division. However, the two divisions were identical, except that students were taught in the first and midwives in the second. He put forward the thesis that perhaps the students carried something to the patients they examined during labor. The death of a friend from a wound infection incurred during the examination of a woman who died of puerperal infection and the similarity of the findings in the two cases supported his reasoning. He concluded that students who came directly from the dissecting room to the maternity ward carried the infection from mothers who had died of the disease to healthy mothers. He ordered the students to wash their hands with a solution of chlorinated lime before each examination.

Under these procedures, the mortality rates in the first division dropped from 18.27 to 1.27 percent, and in

March and August of 1848, no woman died in childbirth in his division. The younger medical men in Vienna recognized the significance of Semmelweis' discovery and gave him all possible assistance. On the other hand, his superior was critical not because he wanted to oppose him but because he failed to understand him. In 1848, a liberal political revolution swept Europe, and Semmelweis took part in the events in Vienna. After the revolution had been put down, Semmelweis found that his political activities had increased the obstacles to his professional work. In 1849 he was dropped from his post at the clinic. He then applied for a teaching post at the university in Midwifery but was turned down. Soon after that, he gave a successful lecture at the Medical Society of Vienna entitled "The Origin of Puerperal Fever." At the same time, he applied once more for the teaching post, but although he received it, restrictions were attached to it that he considered humiliating. He left Vienna and returned to Pest in 1850.

He worked for the next six years at the St. Rochus Hospital in Pest. An epidemic of puerperal fever had broken out in the obstetrics department, and, at his request, Semmelweis was put in charge of the department. His measures promptly reduced the mortality rate, and in his years there, it averaged only 0.85

percent. In Prague and Vienna, meanwhile, the rate was still between 10 and 15 percent. In 1855 he was appointed professor of obstetrics at the University of Pest. He married, had five children, and developed his private practice. His ideas were accepted in Hungary, and the government addressed a circular to all district authorities ordering the introduction of the prophylactic methods of Semmelweis. In 1857 he declined the chair of obstetrics at the University of Zürich. Vienna remained hostile toward him, and the editor of the Wiener Medizinische Wochenschrift wrote that it was time to stop the nonsense about the chlorine hand wash.

In 1861, Semmelweis published his principal work, *Die Ätiologie, der Begriff und die Prophylaxis des Kindbettfiebers* (*The Etiology, Concept, and Prophylaxis of Childbed Fever*). He sent it to all the prominent obstetricians and medical societies abroad, but the general reaction was adverse. The weight of authority stood against his teachings. He addressed several open letters to professors of medicine in other countries but to little effect. At a German physicians and natural scientists conference, most of the speakers, including the pathologist Rudolf Virchow, rejected his doctrine. The years of controversy gradually undermined his spirit. In 1865 he suffered a breakdown and was taken to a mental hospital, where he died. Ironically, his illness and death were caused by the infection of a wound on his right hand, resulting from an operation he had performed before being taken ill. He died of the same disease against which he had struggled all his professional life.

Semmelweis's doctrine was eventually accepted by medical science. His influence on the development of knowledge and control of infection was hailed by Joseph Lister, the father of modern antisepsis, who said, "I think with the greatest admiration of him and his achievement, and it fills me with joy that at last he is given the respect due to him."

So, only after his death was he proven correct! And of course, they then gave him back his doctorate and made him a hero of medicine. But all the way through, he stayed true to his belief and the data that he had collected that other things were killing these poor women. He kept showing the world, and eventually, his work saved millions and continues to do just that. We like to think we are one of the new wave pioneers regarding health and fitness. And we believe 100% we are on the right path for health, happiness, and freedom.

· · ·

Counting calories on a diet will not help you to achieve your ultimate weight loss goals. There are many different types of healthy food and drink to consume while on your journey to lose weight. Make sure you are keeping a positive mind during your healthy diet. Before starting, make sure to have an idea of how much weight you would like to lose. Setting goals before starting a diet to lose weight will help you reach your ultimate weight loss goals. Remember, team, that the weight on the scales is *not* what we are talking about here. For sure, we would like to see the number drop, but only because of the body fat coming off and not water loss, etc., which gives a false reading. As we suggest a few times in this book, we highly recommend using a set of fat calipers because it is the fat under the skin and around our vital organs we want gone! This will then bring us to ultimate health and a more toned figure.

Another thing to do before starting a weight loss program is to go through the kitchen and get rid of any junk food you may have. This will help you not to snack on unwanted foods. Next, make a grocery list every week and only buy those items on the list. It helps to put together meals prior to going to the grocery store, so you know exactly what ingredients you need for each meal. While thinking about the weight you want to lose, you must stay active. Make sure you work out at least 3-5 times over seven days, no more than 20-30 mins with the correct intensity, whether in the morning or evening. Working out for only 20-30 minutes a day can help you tremendously. Keep in mind, just because you are eating healthy doesn't mean you will lose ten pounds right away. However, if you're active, you will have a successful weight loss journey.

Keeping a weight loss journal is very beneficial to you while you are exercising and eating better. Be sure to entirely focus on what is passing your lips with every meal, recording your start weight and body measurements. Like I have just mentioned, an effective way to measure body fat is to use calipers. The electronic ones are notoriously inaccurate. Do all of the above once per month, then, monthly, go ahead and compare your body fat to the previous weeks. Make sure you do different types of workouts each day and change how long you are training, so the body doesn't have a chance to get used to a routine and stop adapting. Our website has all the short workouts you need. Obviously, we need energy to help us burn fat throughout the day, but we don't want to overindulge in sugars and nasty carbs. If you continue to eat lots of refined carbs and sugary foods, the body will use some but store the rest as fat, and you will start to accumulate fat stores. This is why you must portion out the foods you eat and control your weight by being careful of each meal you are consuming. This will help your body to be able to maintain your weight and not store unwanted fat.

And how about this, girls? It's been found that the number of calories you eat does not impact weight loss in the long term. Instead, what can help individuals shed pounds and stay in shape is consuming healthy food that does not contain high levels of sugars like most processed foods.

Now, let's briefly discuss where macronutrients come from and in what form. Carbohydrates come from grains, fruits, vegetables, and milk products, as well as a few other foods. Proteins are the building blocks of muscle tissue. They also provide energy and help to maintain muscle mass during weight loss. Without enough protein, you can't build and repair muscle. They are essential for a fit and healthy body, and having too little of them can cause unpleasant side effects such as increased hunger, food cravings, fatigue, weakness, and more. Another thing to remember is that you should focus on choosing the right foods when it comes to losing weight. For example, if you crave sweets, it's better to eat an apple instead of chocolate cake.

No matter your goal, a great diet helped by exercise is needed. No one denies these two factors are true. However, everyone wants to know our secret. So, what's the secret? Well, the secret is not really a secret at all. It is not spoken about because it goes against everything virtually everyone says you should do to lose weight!. The secret? To learn to speak to your body and for it to understand and then react. I cannot wait for the moment, somewhere in this book, where you say, "My goodness! I understand now!! It is so simple!" Learn the language of the body, and the body will naturally lower its fat stores over a fairly short period. You will be amazed at how cool it is!

If our goal is to lose body fat, become more healthy and be more toned and athletic looking (and let's face it, we all do!), we should focus first of all on our diet. You should exercise regularly and eat healthy foods that are low in carbs and sugar. Of course, it does not mean you should deny yourself the pleasure of eating. There's no reason to go hungry. Just choose the right low carb, low sugar foods that will help satisfy your cravings while at the same time giving you optimal nutrition. Our body will burn its fat stores for energy once "fat-burning mode" is activated, which is accomplished by listening to your body. And, if you follow our advice, your body receives all the nutrients it needs while burning off excess fat. When you stick to a healthy diet and regular workouts, you will see the pounds come off. It's not only easier but healthier as well.

The best way to start your new diet and weight loss plan is by eating "Clean." This means eating food that is as far away from being processed as it can be, like eating meat, nuts and seeds, eggs, great natural fats like butter and olive oil, and above-ground veggies in your meals. All of these are rich in nutrients that are vital for your body, giving the energy it needs to function well and giving it all the vitamins and minerals necessary for bodily health. Don't forget that you don't have to be hungry to eat the right quality of food. Also, remember that it is essential to try the different types of meats, veggies, fish, nuts, and seeds so you can get accustomed to their taste and then choose which one you like best. Let's say you want to lose 2 lbs of body fat per month. You need to keep insulin low by keeping carbs and sugar low. Don't stop following this low carb/low sugar plan when you see that you have reached your goal. Keep on doing it to maintain that weight loss and excellent health. And, by keeping 8 out of 10 meals clean, the meals will be low carb, low refined sugar, and packed with protein. So, no need to worry!

On a slight side note, girls, in working with 100's of clients over the last 25 years, I have seen many over-complicate things. I have tried to "reinvent the wheel" more times than I care to mention, but I have learned everything I could along the way. And each time, I have gotten more innovative and better at my job. Vegan and veggie warriors are fast becoming a big part of my client base, and it is amazing to see. Like I have said earlier, we are in no way trying to tell any of them what to eat. Giving the correct advice to my clients is paramount. Nothing is more important than giving my warriors my full attention and help. So, I would not be doing my job right at all and insulting you, my fab readers, if I did nothing to help my plant-based crew! So, even though I eat all foods, that does not affect my ability to work with everyone. Regardless of what you eat or do not eat, all bodies are the same inside: FACT! So, we all need to be low carb/low sugar warriors for life. The body does not know our beliefs, and to be brutally honest, it doesn't care. All it cares about is staying alive and thriving, So if we deny our bodies a certain food group, they will eventually miss the nutrients from that group, and we can develop chronic issues as we get older. I love the fact that girls and boys, of course, from all over the world, want to abstain from eating meat. I think it is amazing! However, the body thinks it's missing out on key elements and will try to compensate. And it is these compensations that lead to issues.

Moving through this book we will refer to many sources of protein. And, in most cases, I will speak about animal proteins. This is in no way meant to be offensive to plant-based girls. It is just a way of moving the book forward without stating every piece of food on the planet. I am sure you get what I mean. So, to my plant-based girls, you need to replace animal products with non-animal ones. The slight issue you need to be aware of is that to make the plant-based replacements, much refining and experimentation go into most of them. So ironically, even though you are not consuming any meat, you could be consuming a lot of processed rubbish. You need to be ultra-smart with your animal protein swap-outs. But let me make this clear, you can, and will, totally thrive making that one move alone in conjunction with the rest of the teachings in this book! I want to help you discover that companies are still only after profit and have little regard for our health, regardless of what the fancy packet or box may tell you. We need to approach the issue intelligently to ensure our swap-outs are savvy, which we'll talk about in more detail throughout this book.

Mental Hurdles That Hinder Weight Loss

There are undoubtedly tons of challenges that will pop up on any weight loss journey. Physical barriers are very real (being too heavy to exercise as much as you'd like, feeling too large to find comfortable workout clothing, etc.). But the most challenging obstacles to face and overcome when losing weight are mental ones, the ones you create in your mind that scare you into thinking you can't do it. The following are ten of the most common and deeply rooted mental hurdles people use to block their own path to good health.

Please bear in mind that even though I've said these are hurdles we create for ourselves, that doesn't make them any less real or any less formidable. In no way do I want to sound blasé about this. These are the emotional demons that live in our mental closet, all too ready and eager to sabotage our sincerest weight loss efforts. But you can, you must, and you will face these demon hurdles because that is the only way to freedom and health. The weight loss journey is a warrior's journey! A Blade's Warriors journey!!

That said, it's time to put on your ninja suit, and remember, these hurdles are real, yes, but ultimately, they only exist in your mind, and the wonderful thing about a mind is how much it can change.

Lack of Self Discipline

Well, duh, right? Habits are all the activities you do that you don't think about throughout the day. Now, if your habits include getting enough sleep, exercising regularly, laughing frequently, eating a wide variety of healthy foods, and drinking plenty of water, you are in tip-top shape. However, if that doesn't sound like you, you have developed one, some, or all of the following unhealthy physical habits that will sabotage your weight loss efforts.

The walk-by candy thief. That handful of candy you grab every time you pass the "naughty" cupboard; the "occasional" treat from the vending machine that is actually your daily treat from the vending machine; the extra sweets you sneak when you think no one is looking (including that stash of cheap Halloween chocolate you keep in your desk); all damage your weight loss efforts rather quickly.

The coffee survivalist. Do you drive through Starbucks every morning to grab the biggest cup of Joe possible? Do you find yourself shaky without a boost of caffeine before 10 am? Caffeine is a drug and a highly addictive one at that. But used correctly, caffeine is amazing and can help with weight loss. It blunts the hunger signal and can help with our intermittent fasting setup. Adding in black coffee is fab but only around 2-3 cups per day.

To the "just a drink to calm me" guy or gal... Do you come home after a long day and unwind with a beer or six? More than one glass of wine a day will kill your weight loss journey and keep you portly. You might as well be drinking glasses of sugar.

If you have many bad habits (which, if you are reading, I assume you do), you will have to learn how to discipline yourself. The good news is that it does get easier! But you are going to have to fight them at the start of this journey.

Social Fattie

Humans are social creatures. We thrive in packs, and we do best when other like-minded humans support us. You may have good intentions when you're in private, but all restraints go out the window as soon as you go out in public. You associate eating poorly with sharing with people. Eating a salad in a restaurant may seem like you are not getting the most out of a social occasion. It might feel like you are "wasting" the mini celebration by ordering something healthy. It's easier to eat better when you are cooking for yourself most of the time, but if you don't get your habit of ordering bad food at a restaurant under control, eating out constantly will cost you a lot! Try ordering the salad with loads of meat and olive oil on it. It's not as bad as you might think!

You Are Comfortable Feeling Invisible

Most people who have been overweight can tell you that they feel invisible a large percentage of the time, even though they're bigger than the average person (and often the biggest person in the room). It may sound silly, but it's true in the majority of cases. Often, people get comfortable feeling invisible. It feels safer for them not having to fend off people at bars or being talked to by people you otherwise wouldn't speak to. Sometimes it's easier to stay in the fear cocoon of invisibility than it is to come out loud and proud. Some people become overweight because of a fear of being noticed. The fat feels like a security blanket, keeping them safe from predators and scary situations. To be thin would mean being seen, and being noticed means risking being hurt.

And then there's social anxiety, your fear of social situations and big groups of people. Yes, overweight people are routinely ignored, and when you start losing weight, you will get noticed. You will begin to get the attention that has been withheld from you, and it may be frightening or at least disconcerting at first. To combat this, force yourself to get a little uncomfortable (I know, simple doesn't equal easy). That's what weight loss is initially, a whole lot of discomfort. You're eating things you haven't been eating before, and you're moving your body in ways it hasn't moved in years. Why not add the social discomfort aspect to it as well? Put yourself out there. You're a lovely human being worthy of being known. Believe it, and others will, too! But take it easy on yourself at first. You don't have to hit the nightclubs right off the bat. Take baby steps with new social situations. Pick an outing that you feel you can handle and challenge yourself to stay for a certain amount of time, then get the hell out of there if it becomes too much for you.

Let me share a technique that helped one of my clients with a rather acute case of social anxiety. When she began to go to parties with a mixture of people, including many single people, she would get so nervous she'd feel like she would throw up. Then one night at a party she was attending, she attempted to make lame cocktail chit-chat, feeling like she stuck out like a sore thumb, when this little voice inside her head said, "Watch yourself feeling uncomfortable." She stopped in her tracks for a moment. She just stood there, wondering if she could simply observe herself feeling uncomfortable, not judging it, not trying to be in any way different than she was, just observing herself feeling this way. It worked! It took her mind off of endlessly searching for some way to be witty, endlessly judging herself and finding herself lacking, endlessly searching for an exit. This became her modus operandi in all social situations where she felt uncomfortable, and it has made a world of difference. She still uses it occasionally. Please, try it out and see if it works for you. Remember, our minds are meant to be our servants. We weren't meant to be slaves to our minds.

Comfort Eating

Comfort eating is a big reason so many people gain weight in the world. It numbs your brain into thinking everything is okay. We all do it from time to time, but if you are doing this regularly, you need to really make this a priority and fix your emotions. I am very familiar with this feeling myself, and it can be a hard habit to break.

My solution:

Be social. Call up friends, don't be alone. Your body wants to replace that feeling of connection and happiness with numbness so you don't feel the pain. Use that pain! Let it motivate you to change your life. If you numb it out, you are doing yourself a disservice and are taking away a very powerful motivational force in your life that you can use to turn your life around. Next time you feel those negative emotions, be thankful for them and go out and start transforming your life!

You've Stopped Making Progress

When you first jump on a healthy eating journey, you will see a significant amount of progress in a short time.

This is a gift from your body to you. This, however, can turn into a problem later on for most people. If you closely monitor your progress, you will find that you hit plateaus, and you can get discouraged if you don't see results after a good amount of effort. Losing weight is not for the faint of heart! It's hard stuff! Don't let anyone tell you otherwise, but the rewards will surpass any expectations you may have. The solution for this issue is to simply let go of the results and focus on the process. Just enjoy the change you will feel internally from eating a healthier, cleaner diet. It will take time, but you will eventually get there!

You Don't Think It's Worth It

A Little known fact about any healthy weight loss journey is it can be a little boring at times, which is why we have a community of like-minded people on our social media pages and website who are on hand to help. Sure, it's great when you see the numbers on the scale start to drop, and 75% of the time, it's going to be you, with a community of warriors working out, drinking water, and having fun as you see the healthier, leaner, fitter you shining through! But I'll let you in on an even lesser-known secret. The other 25% of the time? You'll feel fan-freakin-tastic! Feeling better, looking better, having more energy, wearing nicer clothes, how amazing is that?

Activeness is just part of the process, a critical phase as you learn an entirely new way of being in your own skin. Activeness is here to stay, so instead of hating it, make friends with it. Instead of trying to avoid it (after all, isn't trying to avoid unpleasant feelings part of what got you into this mess in the first place?), invite it in for a visit. Offer it a seat, make it a cup of tea, watch a movie with it while the two of you hold hands on the couch.

You're Not Confident Enough to Hit the Gym

Let's face it, going to the gym if you're overweight can be embarrassing. For many people, the thought of going to a gym is so uncomfortable it keeps them from ever setting foot in the door. The perceived threat of being stared at by people in much better physical shape is enough to give some would-be gym goers severe anxiety. The truth is, nobody really cares about what you're doing. You go in, do your thing, and people will do their thing. It doesn't matter what they think! Do you want to be fat and afraid, or thin and free to do whatever you want?

If you think this is going to be a problem, here are a few suggestions for you:

1. Get a personal trainer. Sure, if you use our online coaching setup, it's a great value, and it's super effective and worth it. A good personal trainer does not need a gym. They can get you in shape in an empty room or on the street.
2. Get a routine idea. If you show up and have no idea what to do, you are more likely to feel embarrassed. Use our website for all the help you need and see how we can help. Keep it simple and stick to the basics until you have it down.
3. Go late at night. There's going to be fewer people, and you will have more of the gym to yourself.
4. Try getting your workout at home or on the street. Run! Anything.

Just remember, there is no excuse not to lose weight! I did it, and you can do it too.

You Strive for Perfection on Day 1

We've all been there. You think, "Well if I can't make it to the gym today, I'm not going to eat well either!" Or, "I can't afford to buy all organic vegetables, so maybe I won't eat vegetables at all!" These examples sound extreme, but they're nonetheless true for a lot of weight loss journeyers. The problem with this kind of thinking is that it's incredibly detrimental and snowballs quickly into a lot of lazy days and poor eating habits. Even if there are days when you can't get to the gym, you should still eat well. In fact, you should probably eat better on these days than any other since you won't be able to burn off any ingested indiscretions. Even if you can't afford all organic vegetables, you should still consume veggies over processed snacks. Get out of the black and white mindset and get acquainted with shades of gray. Your midsection will thank you!

And don't be surprised to find that when you lose weight, gain energy, fit into your clothes better, and enjoy food more, you also start developing higher standards for the food that you choose to put into your body. Being overweight and unhealthy is a lot like being in a coma (a food coma): the denial required to maintain that state means you shut or block out any input that doesn't agree with your modus operandi of Eat, Sleep, Eat. As you begin to shed pounds and confront long-dormant feelings, fears, and (gasp!) dreams of the life you've always wanted to live but didn't believe you could because of your weight, you begin to wake up from your sleepwalking state and see things with more clarity.

Whereas before your weight loss, eating fast food hamburgers topped with "processed cheese food product" may have been perfectly acceptable. Now that you are no longer a food-consuming zombie, you're awake, and you crave homemade, hormone-free beef smothered with organic cheese from your local dairy. Still a cheeseburger, but the quality has vastly improved. You care about quality now that you're awake and aware. You care about yourself, so of course, you care about the quality of your food. In fact, you may be shocked by what you begin to care about now that you have the energy to care. As you shed your shield of fat, the beauty, variety, and richness of the everyday world will start to show it to you. Choosing to be healthy has required you to admit to something huge that you have worth and deserve to live a long, healthy life. Once you can see your own inherent worth, you will begin to see the value of the world around you.

. . .

Feeling Down on Yourself and Having a Pity Party

Poor me! I've gained this weight, and now I'm all alone, and nobody loves me! That's literally what would go through my clients' minds all the time. She would sit in her office on weekends and use that time to feel bad about herself. Maybe you weren't as bad as she was, but if you were, then I know that feeling. First of all, realize that you can fix this, and there is a light at the end of the tunnel. Many people have done this, and if you stick to the plan I'm giving you here, you will succeed! You can have a normal, successful, and happy life!

You're Watching How Others Are Doing

We all do it. You're sitting there enjoying a coffee, and in walks someone of your relative age. You're sizing them up internally, assessing what good points you have that they don't, and vice versa. Stop doing this.

Comparison is the thief of joy! If you're always comparing yourself to others, you'll never see yourself as the unique and awesome person you are. Rather than comparing yourself to someone else, celebrate your differences. Enjoy that you have fantastic hair and the girl across the way has pretty eyes. It doesn't hurt to be positive about the way others look as well as accepting yourself as-is!

It's true that when it comes to weight loss, mental hurdles are incredibly hard to overcome. Sometimes it may feel like you're standing at the entrance to a dark and scary tunnel. You know that health and losing weight is on the other side, but you can't see them because of all the mental obstacles blocking the way. The difficult news is that the only way to the light at the end is straight through the darkness of the tunnel. The only way out is through it. The good news is that there is a long line of fellow journeyers reaching back through time who have made this journey before you, using our online training programs and nutrition advice! Take strength from their fearlessness and use it to bolster your courage as you take your first tentative (or bold!) steps into the unknown. On your way, remember to laugh at yourself. Take help when it is offered. You can do this. You *are* doing this.

So, as you can see, girls, I have listed a lot of issues that I have seen and heard over many years in the fitness industry that directly affect the ladies and hinder progress. Check yourself to see if you have fallen foul to any, or indeed, all of them.

Key points to take away:

- Have the right mindset from now on, girls! Set yourself up to win!
- DO NOT Listen to the Dogma girls! Make up your own mind.
- Change all of the areas that affect you on our list of mental hurdles.

In the next chapter you will learn....

Do 3500 Calories really make 1 pound of fat? We think not! Let us discover together why...

---

1. Born July 1, 1818 in Buda, Hungary, Austrian Empire (now Budapest and Hungary), and died August 13, 1865 in Vienna, Austria.   https://www.britannica.com/biography/Ignaz-Semmelweis.

REASON TWO: 3500 CALS DOES NOT = 1 POUND FAT

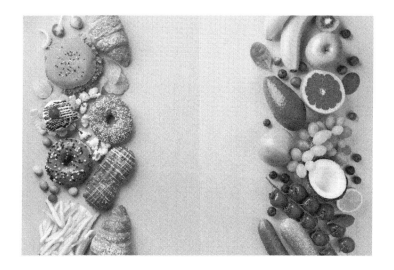

A SIMPLE CALCULATION is used to forecast Calories In = Calories Out. A very plausible and simple calculation in almost every health and fitness publication, yet *no one* knows where this comes from! Not even the top experts! Everyone knows it's right? Dogma in the fitness industry at work again.

Dr. Zoe Harcombe states in her book, *The Obesity Epidemic*, that not only is the following formula incorrect, but she can NOT find any evidence from ANY health and fitness or diet and nutrition organization that supports it! And yet, almost ALL diet books are based upon this one calculation:

3500 Cals = 1 pound of fat (so the Dogma tells us, right?)

So, to lose 1 pound per week, the following formula is used:

3500 Cal - 500 Cal = 3000Cal (Cut 500 calories from your diet each day)

-500 Cals x 7 days = 3500Cal's = 1 pound of fat lost in a week's time

---

And yet, there is no science to back this up. Despite this, almost everyone in the diet world uses this formula for their clients or readers, and after only a small amount of weight loss, the weight goes right back on. Is there not something wrong with this picture?

When people push back saying, "Well, when I cut calories, I lost some weight!" It is very easy to answer, and I always reply with, "When cutting your 500 Calories, what foods did they come from?" Because we instinctively know that if we take a close look at our food, the crisps and chocolate need to come out! You cannot tell me you look at your meal and say, "I need to cut calories, so ill take off the chicken breast and leave on my plate the ketchup and chips as there are fewer calories?" Come on! We are not that stupid, right?

We know that sugar and refined products are bad for us! We know!

So, those are the foods we remove first. It's not the calories in those foods that matter, but the types of foods we consume. The hormonal response to those foods is all we need to be concerned about, not their caloric number.

And moving forward, several more incorrect assumptions are put in, such as the idea that calories in and out are unrelated. We also believe that eating is a deliberate act in which hunger plays only a minor part.

Hormones regulate every aspect of the human body. These hormones control height gain, blood sugar levels, sexual development, and body temperature. The list goes on and on. Nutritionists say, "Calorie fixation was a fifty-year dead end. A calorie is a calorie indicates that the total caloric intake is the only essential variable in weight growth." The hormone insulin VERY MUCH regulates fat cells. Proteins, lipids, and carbs all provide energy to the body, but their metabolic processing differs significantly. Amino acids, which are utilized to create and repair the body's tissues, are formed when proteins are broken down. Carbohydrates are absorbed straight into the body.

Here is some fascinating information about "undereating" or "cutting food" as a way to lose weight. A study was conducted under very tight rules so no one could cheat. Here's what happened...

The Minnesota Starvation Experiment was the world's first hunger experiment. From an initial caloric expenditure of roughly 3000 calories to approximately 1950 calories, participants' overall energy expenditure dropped by a startling 30%. There was no link between calorie restriction and weight loss or recovery, according to the researchers. Dr. Keys conducted an experiment in which he asked men to endure a month of continual cold. The males underwent significant physical and psychological transformations. Even Dr. Keys was taken aback by the experiment's difficulties. The participants had "a very challenging experience," he said.

When men's calorie intake was lowered by 40%, they lost their hair and nails. Except for food, the males were utterly uninterested in anything. They were troubled by continual, unrelenting hunger, and some dropped out of university. The physical endurance of the men was cut in half, and their blood pressure was reduced by 20%. The body shuts down when it is under a lot of stress. It implements energy production reductions across the board to preserve itself. The critical thing to remember is that doing so ensures the individual's survival. You may be miserable, but you will live to tell the tale.

To meet the lower calorie intake, the body must cut its caloric expenditure. Metabolism drops almost immediately and lasts for a long time as a result of calorie restriction. The Minnesota Starvation Experiment predicted a loss of 78 pounds (35.3 kilograms), but only 37 pounds were lost (16.8 kilograms). The return of a woman's weight is not a sign of failure. It is to be expected! Over the last 100 years, everything detailed in this account has been carefully documented! Only a person's mindset toward eating less than 2000 calories per day can improve their body.

"Caloric restriction and portion control simply make you weary and hungry," writes the author. He claims that theories claiming that lowering calorie intake leads to lower caloric expenditure are erroneous. "All we can do now is hope that this method will succeed this time." For the largest, expensive, ambitious, and magnificent nutritional research ever conducted, the National Institutes of Health recruited nearly 50,000 postmenopausal women. The Women's Health Initiative Nutritional Modification Trial is widely regarded as the most significant dietary study in medical history.

The *Eat Less, Move More* diet was given to a group of overweight women. They lost about 4 pounds in the first year, but they were back to their previous weight at the end of the trial. Over 7.5 years, researchers discovered no significant differences between the two groups. Are calorie-restricted diets effective? No. In the Initiative for Women's Health Changing Your Diet, the trial's outcome was a resounding rejection of that technique. Eating less and moving more does not result in weight loss. Instead, it increases weight.

There was no link between calorie restriction and weight loss in this trial.

When the body loses weight, hormones that drive appetite increase. Ghrelin levels, a hormone that makes us feel hungry, rises when we lose weight. This reaction has the desired result for preventing us from overeating. Hormonal changes affect practically everyone daily. The Minnesota Starvation Experiment, conducted by Dr. Keys, was the first to establish the effect of "semi-starvation neurosis." People who lose weight fantasize about food, stress over food, and lose interest in everything else. To obtain more food, hormonal hunger signaling is boosted quickly and indefinitely.

Weight loss leads to a slower metabolism and more hunger, not the other way around. The cycle has been scientifically proven, and its truth has been fashioned in millions of dieters' tears. "We eat too much because our own brain pushes us to," says a dietitian. "Low-fat, low-calorie diets have already been demonstrated to fail." Eating fewer calories does not result in long-term weight loss. "Eating Less" is ineffective.

Now, think of it this way, if we are told to "eat less and move more" and told "that we are suffering from gluttony and sloth," will that fix the obesity epidemic? Then, answer me this...

Tomorrow evening, at your house, there is a huge meal planned. A top chef has offered to come over and cook five superb courses for you and a group of friends! WOW! How nice does that sound? You are told that it will be one of the best meals you have ever had and are advised to bring your appetite! Come ready to enjoy!

What would you do the next day to ensure that you came hungry?

Well, maybe you would get another gym session in? Or walk the two-mile drive to work, and back that day? You maybe even skip lunch to "build up your appetite" for the meal?

BUT HOLD ON! - The advice that the weight loss experts and Doctors are giving to overweight and unhealthy people to lose weight is the EXACT same thing we would do to ourselves to MAKE SURE we came hungry and were able to eat more of that fantastic evening meal!

So, in fact, eating less and moving more DRIVES people to eat more! And it makes us almost obsessed with food!

We instinctively know that eating less and doing more will make us more hungry, yet the experts give us this advice! They say, "Stop being fat, greedy, and lazy, and just move more and stop eating!"

WOW! That's easy, right? No, it is NOT! The body is sending out powerful hormonal signals to keep eating because of the high sugar and refined garbage consumed. The heavier person is powerless to resist and ends up on a downward spiral. Now, I am not saying that the person is blameless, not at all! For sure, better choices could have been made, but we will give you girls all the help we can in this book! What you need is the power and tools to discover the freedom of better food.

What needs to happen is to feed our bodies with the best, most nutrient-dense, high-quality food we can. By the very definition of this one move, this food will be low in refined carbs and sugar but high in good fats and protein! The hunger hormone will feel satiated and avoid sugar spikes! Loads of energy will flow through us too!

So, as you can clearly see, girls, if the modern-day diet books and experts all say the same thing, that is powerful Dogma indeed! However, when asked where this calculation came from or proof that it is correct, absolutely NO ONE can do either of those things? How strange, right?

Key Points - Proving any theory is needed, so prove it!

- Eating less and moving more is absolute rubbish advice to lose weight!
- Restricting food will make you more hungry!

In the next chapter, you will learn some very smart but simple tricks and hacks to make your plate of food better! Simple!

REASON THREE: MINDFUL EATING

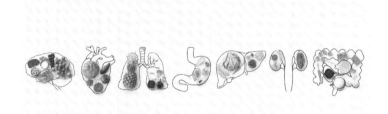

Ensuring You Always Make Healthy Choices

ONE OF THE most interesting things about "diets" is that they're so restrictive. Psychologically, it's disabling. It prevents you from getting where you're going or want to be. We prefer to call it a "lifestyle change" rather than a diet. When you have a scarcity mindset, you tend to hold on to things too much or let go too easily. Neither extreme is helpful for anyone. One of the things that I want to cover with you is mental framework. While we're in this book, and even after, these mental frameworks will be the foundation of your healthy eating habits and getting the body you want. These are simple guidelines that will help you stay away from yo-yo or binge-eating patterns. They're also going to help you feel okay about going off course sometimes, whether intentionally or when you fall off the tracks.

The most crucial part of any lifestyle you lead is to have a North Star to guide it. That doesn't necessarily mean that you have to take the exact footsteps and path as everyone else, but you know the general direction. It's important because a lot of people have very different lives. And we all don't fall into one prescriptive bucket where we can follow the exact steps to get there. Instead, we'll have a general direction that makes us flexible on the journey but eventually end up in the same spot.

Focusing On Inclusion, Not Exclusion

Most diets limit the amount of food you can eat and the number of calories you can consume. You can't eat carbs. Don't eat fat. Drink just this juice. The list goes on. Our program is not going to be a 30-day makeover. Or even 60 days. Or even 90 days. It's going to be a lifestyle. And the reason for this is because you're going to be able to eat most of the food you enjoy. We'll be looking at diets under the lens of what you eat regularly. In other words, your eating habits. Worrying about what not to eat is a mindset that is counterproductive to your goals. Instead, focus on eating the right things often and include foods you enjoy, even those that are bad for you, every once in a while.

Focus On the 80/20 Rule

As a society, we're overly focused on going 110% all the time. We go hard when we start a diet or when we start a workout routine. An all-out blitz initiates any significant change in our life. The result is a failure in the end. An Italian economist named Vilfredo Pareto saw in 1906 that 80% of the land in Italy was owned by 20% of the population. What was even more interesting was that this principle didn't apply to just Italian landowners but business and even nature.

We can take this same principle and apply it to our eating habits. Everyone goes on these radical diets for weeks or maybe even months at a time, depriving themselves of food they enjoy. One slip-up comes along, and it's a crash and binge. Applying the 80/20 rule to your diet, however, means that you can slip up. That it's okay. That's part of the system that we're going to be creating a little later. An example is having a cheat meal.

This means eating stuff that you enjoy, including things that aren't necessarily good for you. At the end of the day, you only live once. Enjoy it. Eating something bad one day doesn't mean your health will suffer. It's just one time you decided to enjoy something a little naughty, and then you hop right back into eating right. The goal here is to live a long, full life. If you have too many drinks at a party, a fantastic ice cream cake for your birthday, or too many chips while watching Netflix, don't worry. I, too, have done all of these things. I try to eat right the majority of the time and work out to ensure that if I do live a long life, it's a quality one. But there are diminishing returns. If I make it to 100 and not 105 because I overate ice cream or burgers, I won't be crying about it, which leads me to probably one of the most important things of all, how you view your body.

At the beginning of my health and fitness career, I used to use this analogy to help explain to clients how important it was to protect your body and ensure your health by consuming the correct food and drink. I'd ask my clients to imagine a machine in their basement just printing money every day. I'd ask my client, "If you had that machine, you'd do everything you can to protect it and make sure that it works correctly. You'd even have that machine covered in case something happened to it to make sure that you would continue to get money. Is that right?" Everyone would nod their heads and agree. Who wouldn't? It's printing money.

The machine is your body. Your body gets you to work and earns you a living. We're focused on saving up for a house, vacation, cars, and retirement. It's all these things that we are saving up for and investing in to live a comfortable life in our later years. But what about our health? That's right. We never invest in it. And if you look to any successful person and ask them what the most critical thing is besides time, they'll say, "Your health." Fueling your body correctly is a long-term investment ensuring that you're going to be comfortable and functional in your later years. And the best time to start? Yesterday. But since we can't go back in time: now.

They say that 80% of health care budgets are spent in the last 20% of life, so that must mean that by the time we have retired and maybe can explore and do more stuff, we may be too ill to do them! And what a shame that would be! Girls, we have to be smart here and see the long game. And remember, chronic illness is not exclusively for 75-year-olds and above, oh no! I have worked with 20-year-olds with liver damage caused by excess sugars! So please do not be foolish regarding your health! Let us help you become bulletproof, ladies!

Set Small Goals, Not Big Ones

Many people have lofty visions when it comes to setting goals, which isn't a bad thing. It's good to have a lofty goal. It's also important to understand that it might take a while to achieve, or it might not be realistic to achieve in a certain period. For example, if you're overweight by 30 lbs. and expect to have a six-pack within a month, that's lofty. Great goal. But is it realistic to achieve in a month? Not so much. Now, this comes in many forms. Some people are frustrated that they don't see results soon enough or don't see the results they want to see when they want to see them. Then they get discouraged and fall back into what they were doing before. This eliminates any progress they made. So, when you're setting your goals for this system, my advice is, don't set big ones. Instead, focus on small ones. Small and easy, and build on them as time goes on.

An excellent example of this is strength training. When I train my girls using the Olympic lifts, we start with a broom handle or plastic tube! Once the technique is locked in, we progress up the loadings, gradually getting stronger over time. We start with a certain amount of weight and do a certain amount of reps. Once my client can complete reps at a certain weight, we add a minimal amount of weight, like 2 lbs., and then start over and continue to rinse and repeat. Focus on the process of taking small steps, and they'll compound. Focus on the small goals instead of the end goal in and of itself. Work at something that is going to get you more toward a more consistent and healthier diet. People who look like they're physically fit didn't dream about it. They woke up every day, worked out, and ate right, day-in, and day-out. The results of these processes are what you see. And those processes begin with small steps. Want to lose 30 lbs.? Cool. Here's one small thing you can do that requires almost no effort.

Tracking

Goals are interesting because you'd think that when you have a lofty goal or any goals for that matter, they will motivate you to keep going. However, this isn't true. Lofty goals put you in a mindset where you're able to push them off until "tomorrow." I've been guilty of that myself. Small goals accomplished over time guarantees a process that determines a successful outcome. Committing to an approach will work. One of my friends was struggling to kick a Starbucks Frappuccino habit. Instead of just going cold turkey, try dropping the added sugar or pumps of syrup. Do that in week one, and then take more off the table in week two. It will be easier to kick that morning habit slowly but surely, and the results will be achieved without even thinking about it.

The sweet taste of sugar is something you can learn not to miss. Reduce the sweet taste slowly, and after a while, you won't even notice it has gone! It will even start to be unpleasant in time. Remember, we can learn and unlearn anything or indeed any behavior; we just need to begin the process of weaning ourselves away from it. Then, when we have that cake or sweet drink on occasion, it tastes amazing, and we appreciate it much more! This is for your health, girls! It is far more important to ditch the sugar for that one reason alone.

Results Are Always Incremental at First, Then Exponential.

I love seeing these advertisements for diets around seasons like summer or the holidays. A diet promising that you'll see results in 30 days before beach season! You do see results, but it comes with a price tag. That price is the strict exclusion of calories or certain food groups, paired with physically demanding workout plans. It's not fun. Like any investment, it takes time to see growth and results. You'll have to front-load the work, understanding what triggers you to eat at certain times, if it's bad food or not, and more. But the work you put in upfront means that you'll never have to do it again. Ever. And if you do have to make changes, they will be minor tweaks. That's the beauty of systemizing things.

This sounds super simple, and it is. But the reality is that not a lot of people apply it in their lives. Even more interesting is that this applies to other parts of your life, like relationships, business, fitness, etc. So while other people go on these all-juice, low-calorie diets for the summer and gain all that weight back in the winter, then go through the same painful process over again the following year, you're going to be in another league. You'll have a system that will let you enjoy the foods you want to eat while still getting to feel healthier, have more energy, and get the body you want. Your diet, compared to others, is going to look a lot like what we're going to cover in the next chapter.

Simple Guidelines

One of my colleagues and a good friend would always talk about fitness, being in shape, and what foods to eat. We'd always talk about people who would ask us how to eat healthily. And it seems so simple, but it never occurs to most people when they want to start eating healthier. It's hands-down the most concise answer to the question of how to eat healthily. It's the simplest seven words you'll ever hear:

Don't Eat Like a Twelve-Year-Old

I love it. So simple. Because if you're eating french fries, chicken nuggets, chocolate, or sweets, consistently, how do you expect to look? How do you expect to feel? And 9 times out of 10, you'll know if you're eating like a 12-year-old. If you don't, it's okay. Revert to the 80/20 rule. You're still ahead of the game. And if you don't feel like it? That's okay, too. Again, the point of all this isn't to say that we shouldn't eat certain foods, but rather eat good foods more consistently than others. This is a great rule when it comes to eating healthy, but generally, even if you decide not to eat like a 12-year-old, you still might run into some challenges. Nutrition is complex. Professionals in the field are still discovering more about it every day.

Food companies know how to frame "healthy" language in their marketing as well. Maybe you think that you're eating something healthy, but it isn't. In this book, I want to make sure that you take away straight-forward guidelines and rules for yourself. Once you've finished the book, it's going to be very easy to under-stand what's healthy, what's not, and what you're putting into your body. So let's jump into it!

If You Can't Find It In Your Kitchen, Stay Away From It

A lot of people will ask me questions like how do I know something is healthy? Or even worse, they'll think that something is healthy when it's really not. The easiest way to eat healthily is to stay away from processed foods. If your food contains something that you can't find in your kitchen, you shouldn't be eating it consistently. Some examples of processed foods are cereal, pasta, bread, cookies, ice cream, etc. When shopping for food, browsing for a snack, or even out to eat, it's important to know what we're putting in our bodies. And, the easiest way to do it?

Read the Ingredients

You'll notice that when you look at a lot of your regular household snacks, they're filled with things you've never heard of. Peanut butter is my favorite example. Take a look at any major brand, and you'll see a laundry list of ingredients in the peanut butter that make you scratch your head and think, "Isn't peanut butter supposed to be just peanuts?"

That's not a trick question. It *is* just supposed to be peanuts.

Peanut butter is made from just peanuts. Crazy, I know.

If there are a lot of ingredients that you can't pronounce, have no idea what they are, or they sound foreign to you on your ingredient list, you probably can't find them in your kitchen. And if you can't, stay away from them! At least most of the time. The last guideline is my favorite. When we look at diets, losing weight, or getting in shape, we always focus on calories. Calories in and out, burning more calories than you consume, and you've got yourself a winning formula for getting the body you want. Well, not at all. However, there are many apps, programs, and courses created to log your calorie intake. The Dogma tells us to track calories when, quite honestly, we do not need to.

Focus On Nutritional Density and Quality of Food

When most people look at a plate of food, they wonder about the calories that they're consuming. However, we need to focus on the nutritional value of food rather than its caloric quantity. Nutritional density or value means that a specific food is high in nutrients but relatively low in refined carbs and sugar. Another way to look at nutritional density or value is a higher ratio of nutrients to energy within a given amount of food.

Focusing on nutritional density does two things for you. The first is that it ensures that you're putting quality, non-processed foods into your body. The second is that it eliminates having to worry about calories at all. This means no calorie apps, no fitness bracelets, no logging of food in your food diary. When one type of food has a lot of nutritional value, it typically has fewer calories. But as we now know, the calorie number is of no use to us. In addition, it also fills you up. For example, if you compare a serving of almonds vs. a serving of potato chips, you'll notice that each has about 160 calories. But the serving of potato chips has less fiber, less fat, and less protein than almonds. A bag of potato chips is essentially a handful of carbohydrates processed in a factory to taste great.

Delicious, in fact, no doubt, but...

The more fat, protein, and fiber food has, the more likely it will keep you satiated. This, in turn, will make it more likely that you won't eat as much. Now, if you use my example above, it's much harder to scarf down a huge bag of almonds than it is a huge bag of potato chips. Focusing on the nutritional value of the food rather than the caloric value helps you not have to worry about tracking food and calories. But it also helps you to make healthy decisions as well. So, now that you have some simple guidelines to follow, let's dive into knowing more about the food you're putting into your body and where to find it.

The Perfect Plate

I've provided you with guidelines, information on how to understand what to pick from your food, and even some common missteps and fallacies when eating a healthy diet. Now, I'm going to give you four rules that you MUST abide by when it comes to eating healthy. These aren't guidelines; they're musts!

1. Don't Drink Your Sugar!

A lot of people will ask me, "What's the quickest and easiest way for me to start being healthier?" Ironically, one of the most straightforward steps you can take toward being healthier has nothing to do with your plate. It has a lot more to do with your drinking. I'm not even talking about the alcoholic kind, either! Iced teas, orange juice, fruit punch, soft drinks, and more are loaded with sugar that you don't need. When you regularly have these drinks in your diet, you add extra sugar, all of which find their way to your waistline.

Stick with coffee, tea, or water. It's okay if you want to add cream or milk. Diet sodas are okay, at best, but I still try to keep those to a minimum. Try club soda instead. Remember the story about my friend who was trying to kick their Frappuccino habit? She would get a Frappuccino every morning at Starbucks. It was a frustrating process to overcome the urge to drink the Frappuccino because it was a daily habit that had been a part of her routine for years. Look, you're not going to win the war in a day. Set small goals. One day, you can ask to cut the number of pumps of syrup in the Frappuccino in the morning. Then next week, take them out completely. Then the following week, get rid of the whip cream or chocolate. Hopefully, you're picking up what I'm laying down. It's a gradual process that doesn't happen overnight. The point is to keep getting after it, and it will come.

2. Eat Above-Ground, Green, Leafy Vegetables, and have Plenty of Protein

It's a foolproof way to always make sure you're eating healthy. There are numerous studies, documentaries, books, and overall evidence that plant-based diets are extremely beneficial toward our health. And we fully support the concept that eating veggies are superb for our health. However, we must ensure we have adequate protein and essential amino acids that would be missing from our diet if we eat only vegetables. We can, of course, supplement these if we do not consume animal products. It's not up for debate among health professionals. In fact, it's not argued about or even speculated on. It's accepted as fact. Eating vegetables is something that you can do to ensure you're always eating healthily. Not only does the fiber in vegetables fill you up, but it helps your digestive health too. So, whatever you have on your plate, make sure you've got greens with it. We advise topping your fab pile of veggies with lots of cheeses and oils! You will get a lot of the missing stuff by making that one move alone! Of course, vegan cheese is all good too!

3. Limit Carbs and Sugars

However, you should try to keep them at a minimum. Carbohydrates and sugar provide you with some instant energy. A surplus of energy gets stored as fat. The reality is that most people don't need that extra energy from consuming a lot of sugar and carbohydrates. Unless you're a professional athlete or are doing heavy physical labor, and even then, I would beg to differ as more energy can be derived from fat burning, you probably don't need the extra energy. If you're reading this, you're a knowledge worker who's sitting at a desk, in front of a computer, or interfacing with people for a large part of your day, then consuming lots of food is not the best idea. Usually, it is boredom or habit that makes us pick up food at work. Try drinking more water or have a black coffee. The hunger feeling can be dehydration giving the same signals? So drink up!

And for you knowledgeable workers, ever wonder why you get that 2 pm feeling after you eat lunch? It might be because you're eating too many refined carbs. Carbohydrates and sugars, especially from processed sources, affect your mood, focus, and energy levels. When you eat too many refined carbohydrates, it causes a spike in your blood sugar and triggers a significant spike in insulin. Cortisol is released, constricting blood flow to the brain, making you feel tired and foggy. As busy professionals who use their intellectual capital to earn a living, it's best to stay away from excessive carbohydrates and sugars because we don't expend enough physical energy to justify doing so. Athletes, physical laborers, or other professions or hobbies that require heavy physical demands may be able to get away with more carbs in their diet. Either way, we have to tailor our eating habits accordingly.

One Caveat is to remember that even if you feel you "need" the extra carbs to, let's say, run a 1ok race the next day, it is not such a great idea to push lots of carbs through your system, regardless of if you can deal with them or not. This again raises the point that the body's preferred fuel source is fat. However, the fat will not be used if the body has carbs and sugar to burn first. We cannot override this! And the crazy thing is that once the body burns its fat for energy, it has WAY more energy anyway! And, it lasts for so much longer than the burning of sugar ever could. So don't "carb load" before a race. Learn to prime your body to use fat! We will give you all the tools you need to discover this for yourself as we go through this book together.

4. Make protein the main part of your meal

If we start to remove the naughty refined grains and carbs from our meals, our plate can start to look very bare! Because we consume so much of it in every meal, it "bulks out" our plates and fills us up. But this is a fool's game. Start to remove the grains and "white" foods (pasta, rice, potatoes, etc.) BUT replace them with meat, cheese, eggs, nuts, and seeds. Do not skimp either. Like we have already said, do not fear fat! It is our best friend when it comes to feeling fuller and

59

burning fat. It WILL NOT make us gain body fat so long as the refined carbs and sugars are very low. The body will thrive on the fats, giving you so much energy and no spike in blood sugar. Then, at the gym or during your workout, you'll not only get fitter but leaner as body fat is burned off for energy!

Chapter Summary

For sure, girls, a lot of information to absorb here! But, every bit of information is here because it will help you! For over 25 years, I've been assisting girls to become fit and healthy Blade's Warriors!

Key Points -

- The most important thing in life is taking action. Remember the 80/20 rule.
- We do not need the excess sugars in our diets!
- Invest the time and effort into a better you! Your body is the only place you have to live in!

In the next chapter, you will learn how we came to use the word "calorie" and where it came from.

REASON FOUR: THE CALORIE
FORMULA DEBUNKED

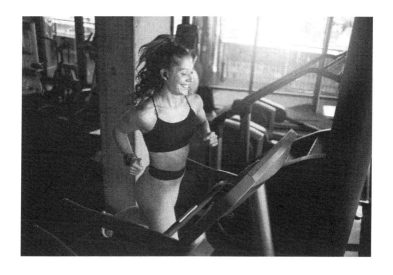

AGAIN, girls, it is time for another science bit! And as before, please read with an open mind as I write down the history of the calorie, where it came from, and why it is so misleading to use when talking about nutrition and weight loss.

"Calorie" is a term first coined in the early 1800s by French scientists working on the efficiency of steam engines. In this context, it made a lot of sense to work with a unit of energy defined as the extent to which burning fuel raises the temperature of water to create the steam that runs the engine. There was a basic flaw in the term, though. "Calorie" was derived from the French word caloric, believed to be a fluid that embodied heat. In other words, researchers at the time mistakenly thought caloric was a substance in fuel that was responsible for the heat output when burned, and calories were a means to measure how much of the (non-existent) substance a given fuel contained. We later learned that there is no such thing as the physical substance caloric, yet the underlying notion has persisted, along with the word calorie.

A chemist, William O. Atwater, cemented the word calorie during his study of human nutrition in the late 1800s. The US government tasked Atwater with determining how to feed workers to deliver the most work output for the least expensive food input. He faced a few serious challenges in completing that task. How would he quantify the energy content of food?

How would he quantify the energy output required for the completion of various work tasks? With minimal understanding of the metabolism available to him at the time, Atwater went to work.

There was only one word in the English language used to quantify energy in the late 1800s, and that was "calorie," so Atwater used the unit in his research. However, he used a bit of creative math to make his research reasonable. Steam engines had an efficiency rating of about 10 percent, meaning about 90 percent of the energy derived from the fuel source was lost during the conversion process, and only 10 percent actually pushed the train. Atwater determined that humans and animals functioned at between 20 and 30 percent efficiency. His observations and subsequent math calculations were based on that idea.

There is a great deal of misinformation in the world. Some of it is based on lousy knowledge but good intention. Some of it is based on purposeful manipulation. Still, more of it is based on once widely believed ideas that have since been proven wrong. The most insidious misinformation, though, is based on corporate profit. Corporations are often willing to sacrifice the well-being of individuals like you and me to squeeze a few more dollars into the next quarterly report.

"There is simply one reason for unhappiness: untruthful beliefs in your mind. These beliefs are so common and so shared that you never think of questioning them" (Dogma!). In my experience, this is true, and calories are no exception. Nearly 60 percent of the world's population is seriously overweight, a number that is growing fast. Obesity has reached the point where the United States has officially listed it as a disability and created a protected status for it. As established earlier in this book, the average American spends the last three decades of their life, 30 years or more, chronically ill, unable to enjoy their life fully, and sometimes unable to enjoy it at all. All of this has led to much unhappiness, and that unhappiness can all be traced to one false belief, a belief so widespread and so commonly held that it never occurs to anyone to question it. You see, there is no such thing as a calorie. In fact, a calorie is not a physical thing at all. It could not be burned even if you wanted to do so.

Let's talk about calories a bit more, and you will understand why I can make such an assertion. Please read this section with me and see what a minefield all this can be! In my experience, people find the truth about calories very hard to believe, even though they see the factual nature right away. We as a society are simply too invested emotionally, morally, and financially in the propaganda we have been taught about calories. Recognizing that it has all been a farce is a hard pill to swallow, but doing so will free you in ways you may not yet imagine. In particular, it will free you for a lifetime of health, vitality, and quality of life.

The Science of Calories

The definition of a calorie is simple (stay with us on this, girls, and hang in there!).

calorie - a unit of measure of the heat energy needed to raise the temperature of 1 gram of water by 1°C.

In nutrition, a slightly different definition is employed, the two technically differentiated by the capitalization of the letter C:

Calorie - a unit of measure of the heat energy needed to raise the temperature of 1 kilogram of water by 1°C (also known as a kcal or kilocalorie).

In other words, when talking about food, we are talking about thousands of calories. That means your Whopper, listed as 660 Calories (big C), when incinerated (literally burned), actually releases 660,000 calories (little c) of heat energy. That is enough heat to raise the temperature of a bathtub of water by more than 10°F!

From this point forward, we will use the lower case "c," "calorie" for our purposes, unless we are listing the caloric value of a substance or referencing a specific source. To avoid confusion, remember, 1 Calorie (big C) equals 1,000 calories (little c).

The critical thing to note here is that a calorie is not in and of itself a physical thing. A calorie is a unit of measure, nothing more and nothing less. As a unit of measure, it cannot be burned. It cannot be held. It cannot be stored. Like an inch or a gallon, it can only measure something else. In this case, increased heat.

Since calories are not physical objects and they are not energy, only a unit of measure of heat energy, they cannot be eaten, burned, stored, or otherwise utilized in any way. This, in turn, means we have all been subjected to a false belief. We have been told that if we eat fewer calories than we burn, we will lose weight. But how can that be if calories are not an object that can be eaten or burned?

Remember how I keep saying that words mean things? Definitions of words mean things, too. If words are used to describe nutrition yet ignore the definition of calorie, they are words that fly in the face of what a calorie really is. It isn't very clear, to say the least.

The Calories In, Calories Out (CICO) model for bodily energy balance does not work, and it never has. Rather than abandoning it, though, the experts try to "explain it better."

When was the last time you heard someone be surprised that "not all calories are the same?" Probably today or yesterday, and indeed recently. They are trying to justify why weight loss happens with some foods and not with other foods, even though the calories listed may be similar. But all calories are the same, exactly the same. A calorie is a measure of the temperature rise when something is burned. The definition never changes, ever. Saying that not all calories are the same exacerbates a false belief. Wouldn't it be better to eliminate the calorie from the statement and simply say, "Not all foods are the same, and the effect of those foods on the body is radically different?" That, at least, would be true.

In order for a calorie to exist, there must be four things:

- Some kind of fuel
- A source of ignition

- Water (or similar liquid with consistent properties when heated)
- A thermometer

The fuel is incinerated completely until all that is left is black carbon. The heat released from that incineration is absorbed by the water surrounding the burning sample. The resultant rise in water temperature is then measured to determine how many calories of heat were released by the fuel.

For a calorie to be a thing in your body, your metabolism would have to incinerate your food until all that was left was black carbon, and you would measure the resultant rise in temperature of your body liquids surrounding the incineration process. Only then would a calorie be a consideration in metabolic function. Of course, you would then suffer body temperature changes of tremendous proportions (remember how an incinerated Whopper could raise the temperature of 30 gallons of water more than 10°F?). You would also poop briquettes, and that would hurt. Obviously, this is just silly. In his book *The Fallacy of the Calorie*, Dr. Michael S. Fenster, MD, puts it this way: "There are not many absolutes when it comes to human physiology. However, you absolutely do not process food by turning it all to ash and naught."

Some still defend the calorie by asserting it does not mean the same thing in nutrition science. It is actually a statement of the energy value of foods and is calculated differently than in other scientific fields. But is it, in fact, "calculated differently?" No. In calculating the calorific energy value of foods, regulatory agencies burn them down to carbon and measure the rise in surrounding water temperature. This is done using a device called a bomb calorimeter, depicted above. To be completely factual, today's food manufacturers use a printed table to determine the caloric values placed on food labels. The chart lists the caloric values to be used for proteins, fats, and carbohydrates. A food manufacturer then determines how much protein is in the food, how many carbohydrates, and so on, adding up the calorie figures from the table. However, the caloric values on that table were all determined using the bomb calorimeter.

As you can see from the diagram on this page, all calories are indeed the same, and they are all calculated using an archaic method that simply does not apply to nutrition and the human body. You might reasonably ask, "How, then, did it come about that calories are an element of modern nutrition science?" And that is an excellent question. To answer it, let's depart from science for a moment and take a look at history.

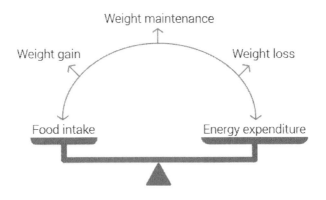

I want you to realize at this juncture that all sciences have long since relinquished the use of the word calorie as a unit of energy. A calorie is a unit of heat released by the incineration of a substance. Each scientific field has since created vocabulary and equations to more directly define specific forms of energy, be it chemical energy, light energy, electrical energy, mechanical energy, etc. Only nutrition science holds on to this archaic and misused unit of measure. While it can be (and is) argued that all forms of energy can be mathematically interchanged, we will see in a few pages why the math doesn't add up when discussing food in the human body. Atwater completed his work under the U.S. Food and Drug Administration (FDA) direction in the late 1800s and very early 1900s. His calculations stand in the FDA to this day and are referred to in FDA food labeling guidelines as specific

Atwater factors. This means that modern calorie counting diets and advice are based on the findings of a man from over 100 years ago! And the fact that these findings have never been tested or questioned baffles belief.

Now for the historical rub. What we know today about metabolism through research in the sciences of micro-biology, cellular biology, modern chemistry, physics, and other sciences began to emerge in the mid-1900s, long after Atwater's research was completed. As early as the 1920s, it was suggested that the FDA choose a different unit of measure for food and nutrition sciences. The FDA elected to maintain the status quo, arguing that the American public was already used to calories in nutrition and would find it difficult to adjust to the change. Today, while specific understanding of the minute details of energy workings in the body is elusive, we nevertheless have a much greater knowl-edge of how metabolism works and how energy is actu-ally distributed and used in the body. Even so, we are still striving to shove the old square peg into our modern round hole by developing ever more compli-cated math equations that simply do not balance.

Macronutrients and Their Effect On Your Body

Your body needs nutrients to grow. It also needs nutrients for energy and to perform other functions. There are two types of nutrients: macronutrients and micronutrients. The former are those nutrients your body needs in abundance to provide the energy to maintain and manage body functions. These nutrients help you carry out your regular activities. Carolyn Cairncross, a nutritionist, states that macronutrients are needed for your body to provide it with the energy it requires to function. Apart from providing your body with energy, macronutrients supply amino acids that are the building blocks used to construct muscles and tissues. You need an adequate amount of macronutrients, vitamins, and minerals to prevent any deficiencies.

The following are the three macronutrients your body needs:

- Carbohydrates (Well, sort of! I'll explain in a bit what I mean)
- Proteins
- Fats

You need energy to enable the growth of tissues and to help in their repair. You also need energy and nutrients to maintain your body's temperature and enhance your body's ability to perform different functions. The energy in your body comes from carbohydrates, fats, and proteins. Macronutrients give your body the energy it needs to function, although the amount of energy provided from each of these macronutrients varies.

Proteins and carbohydrates give your body about 17 kilojoules of energy per gram, while fats provide 37 kilojoules of energy per gram. Your body only needs 4.2 joules of energy to increase the temperature by one degree. Nutritional research conducted shows the proportion of energy-giving food you consume will increase or decrease the likelihood of various disorders, such as heart disease. The great news is that although we have shown the fancy numbers above, so long as we keep up the quality protein and fats while keeping the refined stuff low, our body will get all the nutrients it needs! See, we want to keep everything we do simple, right? So, eating like this will put your body into "autopilot" mode! She will take care of all your needs and wants. How amazing is that!

The Importance of (SOME) Carbohydrates

To be honest, carbohydrates are not all that important. In fact, the body has no immediate need for carbs at all. The brain uses only a tiny amount of glucose which it can manufacture itself using a process called "gluconeogenesis" should the actual carbs in our body run too low. It is a natural system that kicks in when needed. How cool again, right? And yet, all the time, you will hear people say, "You must eat lots of carbs to fuel the brain." It's total rubbish, girls! Once the body has dropped the sugar and carbs from its system, it obtains all the energy it needs from its fat stores. So we have tons of cleaner-burning energy, and we become leaner and more toned in the process! OH, YES!! Carbohydrates in the form of sugars and starches are the macronutrients that should only be consumed in low quantities. When these macronutrients are broken down, they give your body a short-lived energy boost. However, this does not last long and often leads to a slump in performance soon after. We keep yo-yo-ing up and down, which pressurizes the pancreas as it is constantly pumping out insulin to combat the high sugars. The key is to let your pancreas rest and keep insulin release to a minimum. Although a small number of carbs are okay, we want to get most of our energy by burning fat which only happens when carbs and sugars are low, thus keeping the blood sugar low and under control. Protein and fats are of the utmost importance, while carbs are very low on the list.

The Importance of Proteins

Proteins are essential for your body, so include a large amount in all your meals. This macronutrient provides your body with the amino acids it needs. Your body uses amino acids for the following reasons.

Amino acids are labeled as the building blocks of tissues and muscles. These acids produce new proteins that are used to repair tissue and make the essential enzymes and hormones your body needs to support the function of your immune system

They are also a source of energy and the building blocks used in compounds your body needs.

The proteins in your body are made of a combination of at most 20 different amino acids, eight that are considered essential proteins. This means the food you eat should provide your body with some or all of these amino acids. If you cannot provide your body with all the necessary amino acids, you can synthesize them in the liver. Most of the protein you eat as part of your meal comes from animal sources alone. Your meals should contain at least some essential amino acids. Unfortunately, plant sources of protein do not have all the essential amino acids. If you are a fab veggie or vegan warrior, you will need to include a variety of plant-based protein supplements in your diet to meet these dietary needs.

The Importance of Fats

Fats have received a lot of backlash in the last few years, falsely accused of causing heart disease. However, many of the fats you consume are essential for your health and well-being. Nutritionists recommend that you consume enough fats to provide your body with at least 30% of your total energy needs. Fats are also needed to:

- Supply your body with the fatty acids it needs but cannot make, like Omega 3.
- Help to absorb different fat-soluble vitamins, such as A, D, E, and K.
- Add texture and flavor to the food you eat.

There are three types of fats:

- Trans Fats: This fat is found in baked goods, fast foods, snacks, and certain types of margarine.
- Saturated Fats: These fats are found in different foods, such as cream, butter, and meat. Most saturated fats are found in animal sources.
- Unsaturated Fats: These fats are found in different foods, such as avocados, olive oil, canola oil, and nuts.

It is vital to increase the quantity of fat in your diet. Apart from trans fats, which you need to steer clear of, they are all good to go! Do not even worry about the "Dogma" at work again here! The quantity of fats you eat depends on the diet you are following. When you follow a ketogenic diet, you eat more fat than carbohydrates since you need to kick your body into a metabolic state called ketosis. In this state, your body breaks the fat molecules down to produce energy. In a carb cycling diet, your focus is on the number of carbohydrates you eat. So, you need to eat the required amount of fats and proteins to provide your body with the energy it needs. Over the last few decades, nutritionists and researchers have been trying to understand the balance of macronutrients required.

Eat More Fat to Lose Body Fat

When you want to lose weight, you tend to stop eating healthy foods. You try to skip meals and do whatever you can to lose weight. This is a terrible way to go about it since you are weakening your body. The best thing to do is eat high-quality food (satiating, natural, and whole foods instead of refined foods) and reduce your carb intake while upping protein and fat. Also, more exercise goes a long way to help increase your protein intake and maintain your muscle mass. To lose weight, you need to reduce your intake of carbohydrates and not fat. Find the right combination and distribution pattern of nutrients to make sure you can stick to your diet. To keep yourself motivated, you can use a cheat meal once a week as your reward.

Something to think about, If you have over 20% body fat, you should stop analyzing and defining what you eat. Do not overcomplicate the situation, and stop confusing yourself with more information. Eating clean food and being consistent is the only way to move in the right direction, but it is difficult for most people to reach their final destination. As you become leaner, you can adjust carb intake to level out your fat loss. Believe me, if you get this right, you have your hand on the fat-burning dial! Want more fat loss? Turn the dial to lower carb, and the opposite to gain fat. It is that simple! You will intuitively feel what you need to do and when to do it. However, going too low can sabotage your metabolism. However, the body will not use your hard-earned muscle until it has no other fuel source available. So, unless you are at 1% body fat (and let's face it, no one is that low!), you will have no worries regarding muscle loss. The body will simply burn fat and protect muscle and vital organs, so please don't panic! You cannot expect to reach your weight loss goals by cutting your caloric intake. Inevitably, cutting calories is a short-term solution and leads to a considerable weight rebound when you return to your previous eating habits. All the effort you put in has gone to waste. Your body can adapt to different situations, and it will learn to adapt. The effect is that when you are consistent with your diet, you will get the results you are looking for. You can hit a plateau, reaching it because of the hormone known as leptin. This hormone is the satiety hormone, which makes your body think you are not hungry. When you have reduced leptin levels in your body, it will increase your cravings, slow your metabolism and increase hunger. When your metabolic rate declines, it will reduce the energy used, which is terrible for your body.

In addition, leptin controls other hormones in your body. A deficit in leptin can lead to a shortage in growth hormones, thyroid, testosterone, and IGF-1. This is where carb reduction comes into the picture. When you periodically overfeed your body, you have a surplus of energy in your body, which has the opposite effect of caloric restrictions. This eating can increase the quantity of leptin in the body, which will increase the quantity of growth hormone, thyroid, and testosterone. To trim the fat in your body while maintaining your muscles and tissues and avoid all the hormonal and metabolic drawbacks you may face when you follow a calorie-restricted diet, target your carbs intake and decide how to reduce your carbs. You may need to use different strategies to do this, so your body knows how to burn fat to help you lose weight. Then you can bust through the plateau and lose the unwanted flab.

And how about this? Scientifically, "calorie" is a misleading and inaccurate measure of the value of food in the body. Historically, the calorie in nutrition should have died together with the calorie in every other field of science. Even for heat, scientists now use joules, while engineers often use British thermal units (BTUs), both of which are direct expressions of heat and do not require the intermediary of water. Only by the act of the FDA is the calorie still used in nutrition. The basis for its use started from a lack of any other available English word coupled with an inaccurate belief that it measured an actual liquid substance.

Chapter Summary

Whew, that was some heavy science and history, right? But I needed to explain where calories originally came from and how they came to be touted as the only way to lose weight!

Key Points -

- The science of calories is over 100 years old and has not been updated or reviewed since.
- Calories do not even have a place in the modern health and fitness world, yet they stay!
- There are NO essential carbohydrates! Fat is a much better source of energy!

In the next chapter, you will learn why the body simply does not recognise numbers AT ALL, let alone calories!

REASON FIVE: OUR BODIES DO NOT RECOGNIZE NUMBERS

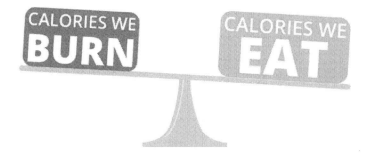

Calories In, Calories Out

OKAY, girls, check this out... Open any university anatomy and physiology textbook, any top-rated health and fitness magazine, any peer-reviewed papers by any scientist, and look for the section where it explains where to find the organ or system in the body that recognizes and counts numbers? Take as long as you need, and get help if you like. Even Google it! Having a hard time finding it? Well, that is simply because NO human possesses one! And yet, we keep talking about calories and counting as if the body DOES recognize them!

It makes no sense, right? But still, the fitness industry and the nutrition guys and girls continue with this false belief that we are some sort of giant calculator that simply subtracts numbers from our food and then burns them off.

I even saw a Doctor on daytime TV mid-way through this year (2021), who, when asked how to lose weight, stated, "Everyone knows that you just do a 500 calorie a day deficit diet. It's easy"! Now, this was a highly decorated and qualified doctor saying it's easy! And everyone knows, right? Well, if it is that easy, why all the obesity? Why are hospital waiting rooms filled with people with problems arising from being overweight? Why are our kids having weight issues much younger? Why is Type 2 diabetes exploding all over the globe? WHY? Why is no one asking these questions? Simple answer: DOGMA! The power of the masses saying it is one thing, and only a few brave warriors standing up to say, "No, that is not correct!"

As previously discussed, the general mainstream paradigm around weight loss is that you need to burn more than you are taking in. As a scientific concept, it's relatively sound, but as weight loss advice, it's horrible. Some of the problems with this model include:

1. It's hard to know how many calories you're eating.
2. It's hard to know how many calories you're burning.
3. It's exhausting to keep track of both.
4. It's so much easier to eat 300 kcal than it is to burn off 300 kcal.
5. A calorie is not a calorie.

1. It's Hard to Know How Many Calories You're Eating

Modern technology thinks it has the answer! But all they did was make fancy gadgets that cost a small fortune and are of no use to us! Also, many apps include a large variety of packaged foods. In theory, you could look up every single thing you eat, mark it down, and at the end of the day, you'll know how many calories you've eaten. But even in a perfect scenario where you keep track of everything, it still gets messy. Just how much olive oil was in that restaurant salad? How many grams of meat? You get the idea. Food is not supposed to be an exact science, so it's hard to turn it into one. Yet again, follow the money trail! Vast profits are made each year selling these products, and the companies are very smart to make us believe we need them!

2. It's Hard to Know How Many Calories You're Burning

Again, the geeks make us think that they have the answer! Most smartphones will track your steps, and based on your weight, they can give you a rough estimate of your daily calorie burn, but yet again, the numbers projected to you will not be accurate, let alone needed! Again, people are not physics formulas, and everyone's metabolism will be different for many reasons. Remember that muscles burn energy even when they are not doing anything. You can take two people of the same age and weight, but one has more muscle than the other. The muscular person's daily energy burn will be higher, but your smartphone doesn't know that. We'll get into the concept of slow and fast metabolisms in more detail in a minute.

3. It's Exhausting to Keep Track of Both

Yes, calories in, calories out is an insanely labor-intensive way of losing weight. And as we know, it doesn't even work! You're always marking down what you're eating (or looking up what to eat) and comparing it to your daily burn. You notice that you had a 300 kcal surplus for the day, and it's 9 pm? Time to go on a 5-mile run. This is a very stressful way to live, and as we know, stress will hinder your progress.

4. It's So Much Easier to Eat 300 Kcal Than It Is to Burn Off 300 kcal

The "experts" tell us you need to run 30 minutes to burn off one Snickers bar. 300 kcal is very easy to eat. However, people are told that 300 kcal is a lot of work to burn off. There's just no way around this fact. Some weight will be lost counting calories, but only because the food you remove to get your calorie deficit always comes from the foods that have the most significant responses to blood sugar. We instinctively know to remove the processed rubbish! The calories we "remove" never come from dropping the chicken breast or broccoli, do they? It's a hormonal response we need, not a number counting one!

5. A Calorie Is Not a Calorie

In my mind, this is the strongest argument against the calories in, calories out model. Your body doesn't treat calories equally. 100 kcal worth of Coca-Cola will elicit an entirely different hormonal response than 100 kcal from broccoli. Hormones tell the body what to do at any given time, and therefore, it's not much of a stretch to outright say that the calories from Coca-Cola are totally different from the calories from broccoli.

How many times have you tried a diet or exercise routine and given up after some time? How many New Year's resolutions have started with a bang and ended with a whimper after the first few weeks of sticking to them? The real reason this happens is not that you're lazy or unable to keep to a schedule. The real reason is one word: habit. You may decide to do something new or different, but no matter how good it is for you, you'll slowly but surely go back to the habit that is ingrained in you. If that new thing is not yet your habit, you will gravitate away from it. Let's talk about diets first. There are literally thousands of diet plans out there. Some even involve a monthly subscription and send you exactly what you're supposed to eat. But if you've ever tried a diet plan, you'll probably agree that it is tough to maintain. One big reason diet plans fail is that they're difficult. You have to avoid certain foods and replace them with, let's say, not-so-tasty foods. Or it may be too hard because the meals are expensive or difficult to obtain, or the diet requires you to maintain a very restrictive schedule.

If you take a step back and consider it, most of these reasons revolve around you changing something or, more accurately, your inability to change.

What you are actually trying to change are your habits.

Your habits live in your subconscious mind. You make rational decisions and choices using your conscious mind, and you make automatic choices with your subconscious mind. In the long term, the subconscious wins over the conscious, with no exceptions. The same applies to incorporating exercise into your routine. If you aren't used to working out regularly, you will eventually give up and go back to your "regular" or "normal," whatever that may be. There are two concrete things you can do to effect a permanent change in your behavior for the better. One involves changing your habits in a very scientific way. The second consists of making a small and somewhat easier change by actually bypassing your conscious thought process.

Let me explain.

Bypassing Thoughts

Even the simplest decisions can be cumulatively taxing if they require some element of willpower to choose between the outcomes. Imagine that you've decided to exercise regularly by going for a run two days a week. Then, on the day you're supposed to run, you find that it's too cold outside, and now you are thinking about whether you should go out for the run or stay indoors. Now, this may seem like a simple decision; after all, running or not running on a single day is not life-altering. However, choosing to stick with your plan does call for a significant amount of willpower and decision energy: willpower to overcome inertia and the urge to stay under the warm blanket, change into running clothes, put on your running shoes, and brave the cold outside. Another example of this kind of simple yet taxing decision could be whether to eat a certain dessert when trying to adhere to a diet plan.

Facing these kinds of decisions regularly is a burden. When you give in to the easier option (and you will succumb no matter how strong your willpower), you end up hurting your willpower. In a way, it sets up a subconscious precedent. Not to mention the guilt that might come with breaking a routine or eating a sugar-loaded dessert. You can make it much easier for yourself to follow through and go out for the run by deciding on it ahead of time. The night before, say out loud that you will wake up at 6 am (or whatever time you're aiming for) and go for that run. If you maintain a calendar on your smartphone, add an entry to your calendar. Set the alarm if you need to. And now, perhaps the most important thing: get your running gear ready. Ensure you have your running apparel and any required accessories set out: shirt, shorts or pants, shoes, socks, water bottle, etc. Neatly lay it all out so that you can see it when you wake up. In other words, set things in motion. By doing this, you are already doing it, the process has started, and the morning inertia may go away because you are already in motion.

Remember, inertia is defined as "a property of matter by which it continues in its existing state of rest or uniform motion."

By taking these simple actions, you are signaling your intent. Your intent is a superpower. Intent starts in your mind but can shape things around you very quickly. Intent followed by simple, small actions can set things in motion, and the momentum that ensues can propel you forward. Now, when you wake up, swing into action. Action is the best antidote to slacking. One small action followed by another small action always works and sets in motion a chain of events that, with time, can change even the most difficult of circumstances. First, straighten yourself in the bed, then put aside the covers, then step out of bed, go to the washroom, do what is necessary to change into your running gear quickly, and step out, one small action followed by another small action, chop-chop-chop no thinking required. If you follow a series of actions one after the other, you can effectively bypass the conscious decision-making process by using the power of intent and action. And by planning this ahead of time, you will be an automaton executing one action at a time.

You can circumvent that decision process by clearly stating your intent by taking some action the night before. And with some planning ahead of time, all you are doing is executing a series of simple steps, one after another. By doing this, you will not be thinking about the cold or the rain outside. You won't actively imagine yourself feeling that chilly air on your face, and you won't linger in bed overthinking the warmth of the covers that you could sleep under for another 30 minutes. You do not need the willpower in the morning to make the "whole" decision of getting ready and going for a run if you can handle most of that decision ahead of time and set things up for yourself to execute a series of actions. If you pause and begin reconsidering the decision, it's effortless to be overwhelmed by the power of your imagination and begin to weigh the run's benefits against the discomfort.

The USDA recommends that healthy adults get 45 to 65 percent of their daily calorie intake from carbohydrates. This we strongly disagree with! We want most of our energy needs to come from fats. Carbs should only make up less than ¼ of each meal and even then be as unrefined and natural as you can get. Carbs are primarily found in grains, starchy vegetables (such as potatoes), fruits, and dairy products like milk and yogurt. Other foods like beans, lentils, nuts, cheeses, and non-starchy vegetables also contain carbs, but in much smaller amounts. Carbs, in general, are easily digested and broken down into glucose (sugar), which our bodies readily absorb. This fast absorption causes a quick rise in blood sugar and then, of course, the insulin response. Carbs can be simple or complex, based on their molecular structure. Although it doesn't matter in what form they come in, lots of them are not good for us! The simple carbs, such as refined sugars, white bread, fruit, and milk, are absorbed very quickly by our bodies, while complex carbohydrates, like lentils, beans, whole grains, and vegetables, are absorbed gradually, both fast or slow is still a no go! The muscles, brain, and heart all rely on fatty acids for energy. The issue is that because modern diets are loaded with carbs, usually refined, and the body can't cope with the excess sugars, which puts huge pressure on the pancreas to keep up the production of life-saving insulin. If blood sugar is high, the body does not need to burn fat for energy. It will simply keep burning sugar while it is in the system. Put simply, it has to! It is dangerous if left unchecked! True, as we have already mentioned, the brain uses a tiny amount of glucose, but we do not have to keep up the large quantities of sugars in our diet to provide this! In fact, when the carbs are kept low, health improves, and the fat-burning system produces a much better fuel for the brain: ketones. This, the body loves, preferring this type of fuel over sugars.

The Carbohydrates Problem

If Carbs are touted as a "superfood" and should be eaten in large quantities with every meal (or so the "experts" tell us), you might ask why I'm even asking whether they help or harm us? Let's first try to understand why carbs have become such an overused part of our meals in the first place. The reasons are simple yet profound. Carbs are both easily accessible and easily absorbed by our bodies and are very cheap to make. Remember, the big companies only want to make more money. Products are filled with refined carbs for longer shelf life. These products are produced to make more revenue! Period! With scant regard, if any, for the public's health. All of these problems and many more create a situation of overconsumption. Easy availability is a function of carbs being derived from food sources grown on an industrial scale, such as by wheat and rice farms and the dairy industry. Massive industrial production drives down costs and hence makes carbohydrate-heavy foods easily and cheaply available to the masses. Thanks to (But NO THANKS) innovations in high-yield crops and fertilizers, food production has grown at a much faster pace than the human population has. The result is that in most developed and developing economies, we are surrounded by carb-laden foods.

The second problem with carbs is how easily they are absorbed. They are over consumed. Incentives and penalties drive most human behavior. At school, you work hard in your studies to earn better grades, which helps you get into a good college or land a good job. You work hard in your job, and in return, you gain either more money, recognition, or both. Sometimes the incentives are non-monetary, like job satisfaction and a sense of fulfillment, but there are always incentives behind most of our behavior. These incentives drive us to exhibit some behavior over another. For example, a regular study habit is a behavior seen in students striving for better grades. In evolutionary terms, the behaviors that an organism exhibits are that organism's "traits." For example, dogs have an acute sense of smell as a distinct trait, while pigeons have an excellent capacity for navigation. Natural selection incentivizes characteristics that are beneficial for the survival and success of a species. Dogs may have developed their sense of smell to compensate for their poorer vision; pigeons (and some other birds) may have developed their navigation superpower to fly long distances in search of food and still get back to their nests.

However, blind evolution moves very slowly and does not always follow a larger script of any kind. Remember, dogs have poor vision. Natural selection could have optimized for better vision, but instead, it fixated on improving the sense of smell. Also, because of evolution's inherently slow nature, natural selection often keeps on incentivizing traits or behaviors that are no longer necessary. Again, using the example of dogs, pet dogs in urban settings don't really need a strong sense of smell to survive. They might end up losing this trait altogether over a long time. Because adaptation and trait change can take several generations and even thousands of years, it's fascinating to see how human behavior based on evolutionary biology can sometimes work against us in unexpected ways. To understand this better, let's take an example from a business to view the situation in terms of incentives and penalties. Assume that you run a marketing group in a company responsible for sending emails and notifications to its customers.

One success metric that marketers look at for such campaigns is known as Click-Through Rate or CTR for short. CTR represents the number of people who clicked on the message, divided by the number of people who were sent that message. So, if a message was sent to 100 people, but only 6 of them opened the message, the CTR would be 6 percent. Hypothetically, let's assume that the marketing department is incentivized only for high CTR messages. If that is the only thing the marketers care about, they will go out of their way to make an email's subject, tagline, or picture in the notification as catchy as possible. They'll do all they can to spice up the notification and window-dress it, sometimes even saying things that are not entirely true, all to spur the recipient to click on the notification. (Remember, just opening a message will raise its CTR.)

Will the CTR go up? Almost certainly, it will, at least initially. Most people are easily drawn to anything sensational or enticing. If you received a message like "Mexican restaurant offering free meals for one year to anyone who...," wouldn't that be tantalizing? Even if you're not interested in Mexican food, you may be curious to know how someone would qualify for free meals for a year! In reality, that message may lead to a survey or sweepstakes. In fact, there's even a term for such headlines or message subjects: clickbait, a (usually misleading) lure for people to click on something. A plethora of spammy websites and emails have these clickbait subjects. The idea is to get the user to click on it no matter how useless the landing-page content is, hoping that some users will stay on the page and click on some ads. This is neither sustainable nor a good business practice, if you can call it a business practice at all!

Thankfully, most real marketers look at many other metrics to measure the success of such notification campaigns. For example, "Was the content useful to the user?" "Did users find what they were looking for?" "Did it help them make informed choices?" "If the page they landed on was selling something, did the user make the purchase?" "How much time did the user who clicked on the notification spend on the landing page?" And so on. In a software experiment, engineers or marketers can quickly adapt and change the parameters of what they want to optimize. For example, if they achieve high CTR but the clicks don't result in better sales or customer satisfaction, the marketers can quickly change their algorithms to generate better-quality notifications by optimizing some other metric rather than just CTR.

Now, back to our nutrition discussion.

Carbohydrates provide quick energy, and those that are sweet provide almost instant energy. In evolutionary terms, this is highly addictive. If you are a prehistoric hunter-gatherer running around seeking food for your family while being chased by a predator and come across a starchy, sugar-rich food, of course, your chances of survival will increase because the instant hit will power you for a short burst of speed. Unfortunately, however, human evolutionary biology has NOT adapted to consume and quickly absorb glucose-rich foods in large and lifelong quantities. Taste buds are very sensitive to pleasure from this fast-absorbing food, the incentive to consume that food. Going back to our CTR example, sweet-tasting, high-sugar foods are like clickbait, giving an instant CTR uplift.

While a sensible marketing team may soon realize the pitfalls of misleading users with clickbait and quickly fix their approach, unfortunately, as we know, evolution moves very slowly. If the evolutionary system has learned to reward a particular behavior and, in this case, reward consumption of a certain food item with great taste and feelings of contentment, it will take thousands of years of evolution to add another "metric" to counterbalance this behavior.

The human body is trapped in an era when food was scarce. In that era of food scarcity, highly nutritious food needed to be quickly devoured. The body is adapted to take any extra energy and store it for future use, not knowing when and where the next meal will come from. Fortunately, food scarcity has been solved for most of humanity, but unfortunately, our biological system hasn't yet gotten the memo. So, here is where the problem lies. We are naturally drawn to high-sugar and carb-heavy foods because they are readily available and lead to instant gratification. This very nature of easy availability and easy absorption leads to excessive consumption without any short-term disincentives.

Chapter Summary

So, Our body has no system or organ that counts! Period! And yet, we are told to count calories as it is the only thing that works regarding fat loss? Well, that's just not true!

Key Points -

- Learn the language of the body - Hormones!
- Eat intuitively. Eat until full. Do not count anything!
- Highly addictive sugar is like clickbait.

In the next chapter, you will learn how to eat to live, and not live to eat. We'll deep dive into our relationship with food.

REASON SIX: EAT TO LIVE, DON'T LIVE TO EAT

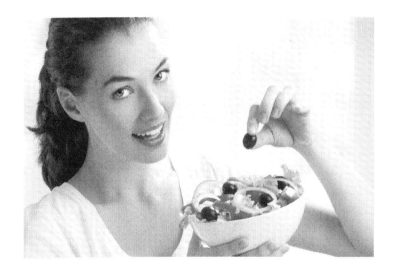

"Healthy life: it's not just about losing weight; it's about losing the lifestyle and the mindset that got you there."

DR. STEVE MARABOLI

AS HUMAN BEINGS, we live in a culture where food represents far more than a source of life-giving nutrition. Food is, for example, an essential part of our social interactions, work functions, and family gatherings. Food is the centerpiece of most major holidays. Eating certain foods is a form of celebration for occasions such as birthday parties and a source of comfort during periods of stress and emotional pain. Finally, the act of eating is paired in most cultures with many recreational activities, such as romantic dates, movies, and sporting events. Living in such a food-centered culture teaches us to use food as a source of pleasure and escape from pain. And when we frequently eat to manage our emotions, we end up consuming foods that our bodies do not need; unwanted weight gain is the inevitable result.

There is only one long-term solution to this source of weight gain: you must develop a food relationship based on well-being, nutrition, and as fuel for your quality of life goals, rather than a food relationship based on emotional management and social and cultural customs. We routinely learn negative food psychology in the world that sets us up for weight gain and weight-related health problems throughout life. We must relearn and replace this relationship with positive food psychology if we are to achieve lasting weight loss success and enjoy the quality of life rewards that healthy weight loss can bring us.

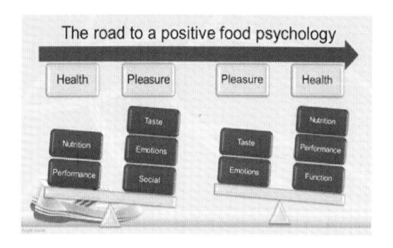

The road to a positive food psychology

Going from a lifetime of basing our food relationship on emotional and social factors to a food relationship based on nutrition, wellness, and performance may seem daunting. The figure above offers a visual display of this change, moving from negative food psychology that produces harmful long-term results (weight gain, guilt, shame, weight-related health problems) to positive food psychology that produces helpful long-term results (a stable and healthy weight, mental and physical well-being, high energy). Based on stereotypes about healthier eating styles, you might currently imagine positive exercise psychology as a prescription for a lonely future eating carrot sticks and lettuce leaves, missing out on holidays and social events, and being forced to give up your favorite foods. That's a very unpleasant image. Thankfully, it is also wholly inaccurate. Consider several important facts about people with positive exercise psychology that can make this food relationship shift more realistic and desirable to you:

1. Everyone eats for emotional and social reasons. Healthy weight people do it less often.

2. Everyone has certain favorite foods that they enjoy. Healthy weight people eat these foods occasionally instead of frequently and better manage portions when they eat them.

3. Healthy weight people enjoy their holidays, social events, and vacations as much as people at unhealthy weights. However, the former group has learned how to make these events less centered on food by developing alternative ways of having fun during these occasions.

The difference between a healthy weight person who looks and feels great and an unhealthy weight person who looks and feels poorly is mostly a matter of degree in their eating habits. Most healthy weight people don't live on deserted islands or subsist on extreme diets to get their results. They don't work different jobs or make different amounts of money. Healthy weight people even eat mostly the same foods as unhealthy weight people. However, healthy weight people consistently practice certain patterns of eating driven by positive food psychology relationships that produce significant differences in their weight over time. Rather than relying on genetic advantages that remain out of our control, positive food psychology consists of specific skills, attitudes, and behaviors related to food and eating that you can begin practicing yourself to get lasting weight loss results.

To embrace the positive food psychology solution, we must destroy the prevailing myth that healthy weight people possess some special metabolic advantage that allows them to eat whatever they want without gaining weight. The widespread belief in this myth holds many people back from developing the skills that could help them succeed. Many research studies have tested this metabolic myth and found it lacking. Take two people of the same size and gender, and their resting metabolic rates will be very close to one another. In contrast to the prevailing methodology, resting metabolic differences between otherwise similar people are small. Furthermore, people who weigh more have faster metabolisms than people who weigh less (not the reverse).

If metabolic rates are about the same, why are there so many confirmed sightings of healthy weight people eating French fries, ice cream, and other highly unhealthy foods without any apparent weight gain consequences? This is because the healthy weight person practices an overall lifestyle where the occasional food indulgence doesn't make a big difference. And because they have kept the refined stuff low in the food choices they made for most of their lives. Of course, this means that insulin was kept low, meaning the body fat melted away as fuel. The "middle-age spread" is a total old wives tale! The real reason for people becoming more out of shape and more metabolically unwell is they are becoming more and more insulin resistant with age. So, going from a 30" waist in our 20's to a 40" waist in our 40's is not because of gluttony or sloth! Oh no! It's the body very slowly being better at storing fat than burning it. I am 50 years old this year (2021), and my abs are all out, so why and how, you may say? Simple, I use our 80/20 rule! I Feed myself correctly 80% of the time and enjoy myself the other 20%.

Furthermore, healthy weight people might eat lightly the rest of the day or two after having a substantial meal or be more physically active than usual. No one gets "fat" from a single meal. If a person eats well 80-90% of the time, the occasional excess won't be a problem. One classic study of weight gain in the 1990s intentionally overfed people living in a controlled laboratory environment for several months. The researchers found large differences in how much weight people gained, despite knowing exactly how much they'd eaten. It turned out that some people became much more active (e.g., walking and moving more) after being overfed, while others became very sluggish. This change in physical activity explained nearly all the weight gain differences.

A second study of healthy and unhealthy weight people on holidays found a crucial difference in behavior that explained most of their holiday weight gain patterns. When healthy weight people overeat at a holiday meal, they quickly get back on track with their diet and exercise routines. In contrast, the unhealthy weight people tended to throw in the towel after overeating and continued to overeat in the days following. This result implies that holiday weight gain is not inevitable but largely under our control depending on how we respond to routine events such as an episode of overeating or missing a workout. If a person who normally gains weight over the holidays begins practicing the eating and exercise behaviors of people who maintain or even lose weight, they will get better results. Despite decades of study and all our high-tech metabolic science, we have yet to find even one of these people who can literally "eat whatever they want and never gain an ounce" or those who "gain weight just by looking at food." They remain the Bigfoot and unicorns of the weight loss world.

Debunking this metabolic mythology is vital because it helps us focus on the positive food psychology relationship that makes most of the difference in the long term. If you are one of those people with a modestly slower metabolism than other people, breathe a sigh of relief that this difference amounts to a small disadvantage that can be overcome with a little more consistency and eating skill on your part. Ridding ourselves of metabolic mythology is also valuable because it conquers the fear that improving our relationship with food requires impossible sacrifices. You don't have to become a health nut, a practicing vegan, go on the Atkins or Paleo diet, or even give up your favorite foods like chocolate to improve your food relationship. But you must change your food relationship in several fundamental ways that involve both learning and practice:

1. You must improve the quality of your food relationship such that 80-90% of the time, you are eating to give your body the fuel it needs to look and feel great.
2. You must learn to recognize and replace the habit of eating for emotional reasons with healthier ways to help yourself feel good and reduce negative emotions.
3. You must learn new skills and behaviors for social occasions to help you live a vibrant life with your friends and family that doesn't jeopardize your waistline.

Improving Your Relationship With Food

The great stories of love, adventure, and success in our culture share the theme of the main characters facing and overcoming seemingly insurmountable adversity. Adversity in these stories doesn't disappear to make it easy for the protagonist; instead, they must rise to the challenge. The hero evolves throughout the story, becoming stronger, wiser, and more resourceful than the source of adversity. Their personal growth is the reason they succeed. This theme of personal transformation triumphing over early adversity applies equally in your quest to develop positive food psychology. Personal growth and transformation are required because most of us are firmly under the spell of negative food psychology as adults.

How does negative food psychology capture our brains? Almost from birth, we are trained as humans to treat food as a tool for changing our emotional state. For example, when a baby cries, one of the most common parenting responses is to soothe them with a pacifier (notice that even the pacifier name denotes the intended emotional response) or bottle. Sigmund Freud once referred to an "oral fixation" as a harmful behavior pattern among adults using infant-aged oral strategies such as eating, drinking, and smoking to gain pleasure and ease pain. As the baby grows into a child, we introduce them to an increasing number of ways to use food for emotional reasons. We celebrate their birthdays with cake, their holidays with sweets and desserts, and comfort them after a painful trip to the dentist or doctor with candy and ice cream. TV exposes them to restaurant advertising strategically linking processed foods to positive emotions with clever labels such as "Happy Meals" and pairing processed foods with popular toys. Escape the restaurant scene and take the same child to the grocery store, and you'll find highly-refined sugar sweets and processed foods virtually shout out to them with vibrantly colored packages and cartoon character spokesmen (e.g., Tony the Tiger, Ronald McDonald, Pillsbury Doughboy, The Kool-Aid Man, etc.). Even if the child somehow reaches teenage and early adulthood in the modern world without weight and body image problems, the negative food psychology training cycle only escalates as alcohol and energy drinks are added to the food-as-emotions mix.

Here's the thing: energy management is only one small function of the metabolism, and providing an energy fuel is but one small part of the purpose of food. So here we go, it's time for another bit of science! As you read with us, think about how important protein and fats are and how little we need any form of carb. Let's take a look at three essential facts about how food is used in our bodies. This chapter will begin to open the door to an understanding of exactly how you can take charge of your metabolic health, including weight loss, cardio-vascular optimization, and total body health. In other words, this chapter will help you learn how to take charge of your wellness.

. . .

Fact #1 - Food Is Your Body's Lego Set

While scientists incinerate food until nothing's left except a pile of carbon to determine caloric value, your body eliminates as much as 20 percent of your food almost immediately. When digestion is complete, there is a mass that remains entirely unused. Of the food that is digested, most of it is utilized in body maintenance. Remember the Legos? Your food delivers the building blocks to your body.

The protein you ingest is broken down into its basic blocks, the 20 amino acids your body needs to synthesize necessary proteins. The proteins in your body are being repaired and replaced in a constant cycle, requiring an endless supply of protein from your food. Of the 20 amino acids your body needs to carry out this task, 11 can be synthesized by your body itself, but nine cannot and must come from food sources. Incinerated amino acids would be useless to your body in this process, right? Although proteins are considered calories on food labels, the truth is that your body does not utilize many proteins as fuel. Instead, they are used as blocks to build, repair, and maintain cell structure. They also communicate important messages throughout each body system and taxi other particles through the bloodstream, to name just a few of their multitude of functions.

Fats are similarly misunderstood. Clever advocates in the food industry teach us that fats eaten are converted to fat in the body unless, of course, we "burn" those fat calories first. Food labels assign fats a caloric value, different from the value attached to protein. Fats, though, just like proteins, are broken down into their smaller particles through digestion, fatty acids, and repurposed in your body. Fatty acids are used in your body for everything from building cell wall structures to acting as fat-soluble vitamin carriers. Fatty acids can be further broken down to facilitate inflammation (crucial for calling immune system help to an injured site), de-inflammation, local area hormone structures, and blood thinners, just for starters.

Ingested DNA and RNA, or nucleic acids, are broken down into nucleotides that will be restructured into nucleic acid molecules consistent with human makeup. Carbohydrates, which you likely refer to simply as carbs, are broken down into sugars, the most common one in your body being glucose. These four groups, proteins, fats, carbs, and nucleic acids, are known as macromolecules, and they compose four of the basic groups from which nutrients are extracted in the body. Imagine them as Lego sets. They are the first things in your food that are identified by your body and broken down into their substructures by means of catabolization. But remember, although the carb (glucose) is recognized along with the other three macros, it does not promote a positive response like they do. The body has to deal with it quickly to stop blood sugar from rising.

In a perfect world, your food would come primarily from plants and other animals. As such, the protein, fat, carb, and nucleic acid macromolecules from your food sources would naturally be configured to meet the needs of your human body. Catabolism breaks these Lego sets down into their individual Lego pieces, and anabolism restructures them into the macro-molecules required by your body. Of course, there is much more to your food than these four macromolecules. Some assert that there are just 11 vitamins and four minerals essential to good health, but there are, in fact, more than 90 essential nutrients that your body needs to survive and thrive. You can easily discern already that nothing at all is in any way "burned" in these processes, right? If the food you ate was burned up as energy, where would the necessary Legos for building the cells in your body come from? On the contrary, the catabolized Legos are needed in their whole, unburned state in order to assist in building, repairing, and maintaining your body.

It follows that your body repurposes the majority of the food you eat according to its needs. This is perhaps the most important piece of information about your metabolism that I can impart to you because it illustrates what you truly must focus on if you are to achieve a measure of health and wellness. You need to focus on the quality and type of Lego sets you choose to provide for your metabolism. You need to stop focusing on calories, which are not even things in your metabolism, and focus instead on the nutrient quality of your food because those nutrients are the Lego blocks your body is using to make and keep itself fit and healthy. These nutrients are involved in every aspect of your existence, from physical structures to spiritual awareness to mental acuity to emotional well-being.

It is time: STOP counting calories and START paying attention to your Legos, the nutrient content of your food.

Fact #2 - Yes, Food Does Provide Energy for Your Body

Yes, your body uses energy. However, it does not come from heat like a steam engine. Instead, it comes from a chemical reaction involving a molecule often referred to as the "high-energy molecule," Adenosine Triphosphate, or ATP for short. We call ATP the energy currency of the body, and it exists in every cell for use whenever energy is required. ATP releases energy when a chemical bond between its phosphate groups is broken. Whenever energy is needed for a process, a protein is broken in the ATP molecule, providing the needed energy. ATP is thus catabolized, or reduced, to a smaller molecule: adenosine diphosphate, or ADP. Now that the required energy has been delivered, ADP needs to be recharged, like recharging a battery, before being used as an energy source again. This recharging is done inside each cell by the mitochondria, which receive the ADP molecule and add another phosphate group via anabolism, turning it back into ATP. The ATP is then ready to provide energy again whenever needed. This process of ATP becoming ADP before being recharged back into ATP, known as cellular respiration.

Cellular respiration utilizes Legos from our food. Our body needs to burn fat as its primary fuel. Carbs are not as important in any way. Keeping them low should be a crucial part of your overall philosophy. Glucose is only needed in tiny amounts. We do not need to take in carbs for this level to be maintained. Our body will create its own glucose if needed. So it is a myth that we must eat carbs to keep up our glucose levels. We need fat as our primary fuel source, made possible by low carbs and sugars. Thus, low insulin = fat burning. Ketones are then produced, which the body prefers as its energy source. At this point, the body needs to live on its own body fat, which is readily available. Fat burning is the body's default state, and it's a myth that we need to exercise to burn fat. The body needs to create glucose from our protein stores.

In this process, amino acids are broken down and oxidized for energy in the absence of carbs. Glucose is catabolized down even further to facilitate the needed phosphate group. Besides glucose, fatty acids can be further broken down for this purpose, and, if absolutely necessary, proteins can also be catabolized for this function. Proteins are not the preferred source for the body to utilize, however. First, glucose will be catabolized to provide anabolism, the necessary building blocks. Then, fatty acids and proteins are used as a last resort. Understanding the actual process your body uses to meet its energy needs tells you something about how you should eat. Certainly, we should not overbalance our carb intake but eat above-ground green leafy veg. These will provide lots of vitamins but have a low carb content, giving you the highest level of health and vitality.

Fact #3 - Your Body Throws Away What It Does Not Need

This fact is critically important for you to understand. You eat food. Your body breaks that food down into its most basic components and uses those components to create whatever it needs to survive and thrive. Your body breaks some of those components down further to provide energy via the ATP/ADP cycle. Whatever is left over is thrown away as waste. And right here, you may again be throwing up your hands and objecting. If your body throws away superfluous Legos, that is to say, any extra building blocks remaining after catabolization and anabolism are complete as waste, why do we get fat? Isn't fat stored energy? Doesn't the body save everything and, if we eat more than we use, pack it away as body fat for later use? No, it does not. At least, not in the way you think it does. There is perhaps more misinformation bloating blogs and media releases about this one point than any other, misinformation leading the public to make very poor food choices. If you provide your body with what it requires and eliminate poisonous substances from your diet, your body will use what it needs and quite liter-ally eliminate the excess as waste.

Cellular biologists learn more about this phenomenon every day. Take cholesterol as an example. Now, we won't get into the whole debate about "good" and "Bad" cholesterol! In fact, all cholesterol is perfectly fine and is once again used as a scapegoat by experts who say it's horrid stuff! More crazy talk! But because the good old Dogma is working its magic again, we all jump on the bandwagon! For clarity, only about 25 percent of the cholesterol used by your body comes from food sources. Your liver synthesizes the remaining 75 percent. If the liver makes too much, the excess is elim-inated as waste. Cholesterol unused by your body's cells is also returned to the liver, where it is converted to bile salts and eliminated in the feces. If there is an elevated cholesterol level in the blood, it is because cholesterol is required to fulfill its primary functions of healing injury and building cells. Excess is always eliminated unless there is a reason for its continued existence. When elevated cholesterol is present, it is more important to discern why the body needs it and address that cause. Taking drugs to reduce cholesterol without addressing the cause of the increase may very well cause more harm than good. So, poor old cholesterol gets a bad rap all the time! When in fact, it is only there to help our cells that are in trouble! It is like blaming a fire truck that turns up quickly to a bin fire. It is there to help. It didn't cause the fire!

Excess body fat is also eliminated as waste. There is no necessity for it to be burned, and in fact, it never is. Excess fat is simply thrown away by the body. If fat is being stored, it is because your body has an imbalance, a state of malnutrition, that your body perceives as a crisis.

Diets Don't Work!

Diets don't work! Google it! At least they don't have a lasting effect. The problem with dieting is that it is a temporary action with a temporary result. Most people go on a diet to fix something wrong with them. Well, I am here to tell you that there is nothing wrong with you! The only reason you think you need to be fixed is that the media and our society have marketed many belief systems, and you bought into them!

The belief system being fed to you repeatedly by the media and through your interactions with others is that you are not good enough unless you look a certain way. When you buy into these lies, you feel bad about your body.

You may think:

- I'm too fat.
- I'm too thin.
- My knees are sagging.
- I have a muffin top.
- If I could just get rid of this back fat...
- I have too many lines around my eyes.
- My eyelashes aren't long enough.
- And on and on.

We can beat up and pick on any part of our bodies we choose, but we got the idea to do so from somewhere else.

For example, you see a magazine that advertises the following on its front cover:

Get Rid of Jiggly Arms

You go home, hold up an arm to the mirror and wave, and then think, I've got jiggly arms, and I need to get rid of them.

You have just been sold a belief.

We acquire many beliefs about our body in this way, and that's just one measly example.

Most people start on the dieting path innocently. They don't intend to make it a life-long career, but what happens is this:

They are unhappy with some part of their body or their weight, and so they go on a diet and restrict their food intake. They begin following guidelines on how they should eat.

Then one of two things happens, or both:

1. They lose weight and go back to their old ways of eating and doing things. Perhaps they indulge a little since they were deprived during their diet and think that they can indulge just this one time since they have lost some weight.

2. They fall off the wagon while they are on the diet, and for all of the food they deprived themselves of, they now eat even more to compensate. They then go back to their old patterns of eating.

In both scenarios, they regain the lost weight, usually adding a few more pounds to their body than before they went on a diet in the first place. Feeling bad about being back to where they were and putting on additional weight, they beat themselves up emotionally for it. They feel like a failure. They feel not good enough, not hot enough, not beautiful enough, and not lovable. Finding themselves feeling unhappy with their body and their weight, they find another diet, a program, or a diet pill to help them lose weight. They vow that this time they will stick to it for good and vow that they will never eat bad foods again. They have a fierce sense of determination and the best of intentions. So they follow their program, take their pills, exercise in the morning and again at night, pass up on the foods they enjoy, and eat what they are told they should eat.

But then, a moment comes when they are at a birthday party, and everyone has cake, or they're at a BBQ serving cheeseburgers, and they say, "Just this once, I'll have a piece of cake," or, "Just this once, I'll have a cheeseburger," and so they do.

Then they feel guilty, that icky, yucky sensation that they are a terrible person and have done something horrible, and now their entire diet is ruined.

So, they do one of two things:

1. They punish themselves. They cut back even more on their food intake the following day, and they throw in an extra hour of cardio on top of the one and a half hours they were already doing.

2. They say, "Sod it, I've already messed up and blown it," and continue to eat everything they think is bad until they are numb from true emotion because they can only feel how full their stomach is. They go back to their old patterns of eating, regain any lost weight plus more, give themselves an emotional beating for failing again and still being fat and imperfect. Until the day rolls around again when they believe a promise from another program, diet, or pill that says all they have to do is follow the program. The cycle continues, and with each new diet, more weight is put on. It becomes a battle, a fight. Diets don't work in the long term for weight loss and happiness, and there are tons of statistics and studies to support that.

What does work? You have most likely heard that a healthy lifestyle works, but how do you know what that lifestyle looks like when you have been taught a million different ways on what to eat, what not to eat, what is healthy, what isn't healthy, what is good, and what is bad? Well, it starts with the Love Your Body Cycle. The Love Your Body Cycle is the opposite of what the media teaches you and what you hear people saying. The Love Your Body Cycle doesn't start with what you should and shouldn't do. It begins with connecting to your body and spirit, communicating, honoring, and being kind.

It works like this:

You treat your body with kindness. You give it kind messages, being aware of your old thought patterns and changing them. You honor your body by taking care of it, asking it what it needs from you today, and then listening to how your body responds. This builds trust in your relationship with your body that is probably not there right now. When you begin to trust your body and your body begins to trust that you will take care of it and be kind to it, your relationship with your body grows. This, in turn, makes you love your body and respect it. When you love your body and respect it, you naturally want to do good things for it. You want to treat your body with kindness, ask it what it wants and listen.

Meditation for a Healthy Diet and Body Image

People tend to blame genes or external factors like eating habits, available food at one's disposal, or emotional stress for being overweight. People try to escape the fact that they are responsible for their eating choices and the quantity of the food they eat. This makes it easy to go back to our original poor eating habits even after starting meditation. However, through meditation, we understand our role and contribution to our journey to weight loss. Changing one's eating habits and patterns is not an easy step and requires patience, motivation, and focus. Always surround yourself with people who can motivate you to make healthier choices. We need not blame our genes but try to work on making better health choices.

I must confess to not really believing in meditation myself until only a couple of years ago. As you read this book, girls, I hope you pick up on the fact that I have always been sincere. If I have been in a situation with a client, or indeed, with myself, I will always let you know! This is critical, as you are embarking on a life-changing journey, and we are your guide! You must trust in us to lead you down the right path. Once I started my daily short meditation window, the rest of my days began to drop into place.

Helpful Tips Concerning Food and Meditation

Go slow with your meals, put more emphasis on chewing slowly, and know the taste of each bite. Treat the moment as if you will describe to someone exactly how the food tastes. Doing this helps you keep the focus on the food you eat and appreciate different tastes, even the unpleasant ones. Create a mealtime and adhere to it. Avoid eating when you are doing something else, which prevents overindulging and helps you measure the quantity and eat to satisfaction rather than leisure. Multitasking as you eat can lead to overeating or indulging in unhealthy foods. Respond to hunger and satisfaction. When you are hungry, eat. Do not deny your body food. And when you are full, stop eating. Listen and communicate with your body what-ever it is telling you and respond appropriately. Know how different kinds of food make you feel after you eat them. Consider which meals make you tired or energized? Avoid food that makes you tired since it reduces the body's metabolism.

Learn to forgive yourself for overindulging even when you are not hungry. The food that you ate made you tired, right? Don't worry about that little blip in judgment, and continue to eat the food that keeps you energized. Understand that you are not perfect and are bound to be tempted to eat the foods you don't want to eat. Remember, we are hardwired to crave the sugary stuff! But we can and will change that! When you give in to temptation, forgive yourself, and move on. Spend time and make responsible food choices. Always plan for the kind of foods you'll eat in advance. If you can't do this all the time, make a weekly or daily meal plan. Acknowledge your food cravings. By doing this, you will resist your craving by understanding that it is reasonable to crave, but you do not have to give in to all types of cravings.

We can design specific techniques and practices concerning mindful eating, meditating, and intuitive eating. By these techniques, we get to have a healthy and productive relationship regarding food and thereby eliminate any bad feelings associated with diet and our eating habits. This result is healthy weight loss. Although this should not be the key focus, it should serve more as a reward. If we focus on weight loss as the primary goal, we may be distracted and not have a focused mind during meditation. When eating, though, you should eat because you are hungry and need to satisfy yourself. Do not eat because you are stressed at work, or have family issues, or as an attempt to manage stress. Meditation practices help you love your body and be in control of your mind and the decisions you make.

General Health Affirmation

General health affirmations are statements, phrases, or words that you use in your daily life. Their main task is to give you maximum motivation in everything you do. You will speak and repeat them to yourself as necessary throughout your day. Phrases like this include:

"I radiate confidence." Confidence refers to the ability to show boldness in what you are doing. You must now be in a position to radiate not only faith but also grace and beauty. Virtues like these are highly significant since they will always guide you daily. You will feel relaxed, motivated and have an urge to be successful in life. Your health improves, and you will be able to see this in your body image. Elements of grace and beauty will affirm you to your real-life situations. You will maintain this kind of morale, which will eventually help you make correct decisions when it comes to healthy food. It is good to assert that choosing a healthy diet is useful to your life and economical. A proper diet, too, results in an accelerated appetite and urge to eat more. Healthy food is always good for your body as it supplies you with vital nutrients. Nutrients have the power to uplift your body, thus improving your body image.

"Every cell within my body accepts good health." Good health will always make your whole body vibrate. It is up to you to concentrate on maintaining good health throughout. You can do this by choosing healthy food from the stores. Healthy eating includes animal products, fats, and protein with low refined carbs and sugar. Vegan and veggie readers need to find a quality "non-animal-derived" substitution to achieve the same goal. The healthy meal plan also incorporates a large intake of water and daily exercise. All these nourish your body's cells, making them carry out their work accordingly. Your motivation to eat every day will develop suddenly, especially when you have all these healthy foods at your doorstep. In the long run, your body weight will reduce due to the assimilation of a healthy diet. And in the end, your body image improves.

You must love and show some respect for your body. Your body is a complex system that needs attention and self-love. Show some love to your body by providing it with everything that it needs. The body needs nourishment, which comes from food. Choose food that is as healthy as possible. Healthy food will offer your body that glimmering natural look. You will also reduce weight, thus improving your body image. Elements of love, respect, and other virtues always act as stimuli that help you achieve much in your body. You will realize that your weight reduces without facing difficulties in the process. Weight reduction will come from choosing wisely the correct diet and using affirmations like the ones above to accelerate their intake into your body.

Another general health affirmation is to be in a situation where you can choose issues like health and wellness and shun or shy off boring workouts, restrictive diets, and so on. I know you might love workouts, but some exercises are just unpleasant. But remember, the workouts completed with intensity and fire in our belly over a short time frame are very effective and time-efficient for the busy lady. Again, there are restrictive diets that you need to avoid. Eating refined foods from packets, completely processed flour, and relying on junk dishes will negatively affect you. You can improve your body health by deciding on a healthy diet. Your welfare, too, is paramount. It matters a lot not only to you but also to your general economic status. Making these choices will accelerate your need to have healthy food at your disposal. As a result, your motivation to eat healthy increases. All these will lead to improved body image with a decrease in your weight. One great move we very much recommend you start to implement is an intermittent daily fast. It is so simple yet very effective in the pursuit of metabolic health and lower body fat. Take a 24 hour day, refrain from eating any food for 14-16 hours, then have your 2-3 meals in the remaining 6-8 hours. So from your last meal in the evening, start the fasting window. As you sleep 6-8 hours of the night, you are already well into the fast when you wake. Instead of having breakfast straight away, hold off for a few more hours, then eat! Your body will have started to burn its own fat as energy. This then strips fat from you AND gives the digestive system a rest, allowing the body to divert energy elsewhere to repair, etc. For such a simple and totally FREE move, it's the best! Plus, you're not scrounging around looking for the next meal! It's so freeing too!

We advise lots of water to help the fat-burning process. But remember, do not diet! Eat well and get all your meals in but in a smaller eating window. Insulin stays low! Blood sugar stays low! Body fat stays low! Energy goes up! It's a WIN-WIN!

Chapter Summary

We must change our relationship with food. We must use it as fuel to nourish the body to do other fab things! Simply put, have a great meal, then get out and rock the day, girls!

Key Points -

- Learn to meditate. It will set up the day and your life.
- Use intermittent fasting every day, girls. We believe it is one of the best things you can do for great health and low body fat!
- Do not worry about cholesterol. It is there to help us. We make it if it is not ingested. So if it is that bad and experts say we need less, why does our body make MORE when needed? Dogma!

In the next chapter, you will learn how vital hormones are in the body and how we can understand them better to improve our health for life!

REASON SEVEN:
BMR/HORMONE/MENSTRUAL CYCLE
DAMAGE

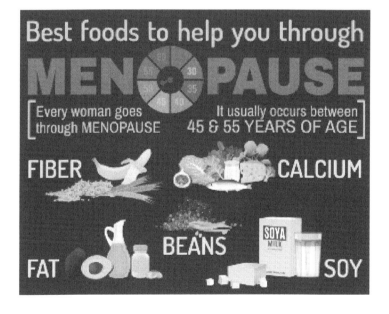

GIRLS, we reach our final reason for not counting calories. And it is a massive one! When we talk about the female body, it is an amazing thing for sure. Restricting food to lose weight puts so much pressure on our health and can even drive some to madness! But a lady's delicate reproductive system is also under huge pressure through this restriction. One of my clients from a while ago (and I have heard about many others since) stopped her monthly periods while dieting because she was not getting enough calories. And, at the time, she was trying to start a family. She was weak and unwell because the dogma had told her to cut calories to lose weight! But there is a happy ending to this little story. After talking with me in detail and then eating correctly based on the information I gave her, she started to gain her health and build quality muscle too. Then, not too long after, she became pregnant! She now has two healthy girls, and she is flourishing!

The overall factor that helped the most was the freedom not to count, weigh, or measure anything. She simply eats well and thrives in life!

We are talking about menopause, girls. Now, please do not roll your eyes. You may very well be a younger girl reading this thinking, "This doesn't affect me; I'll skip this part." However, please bear with me. Through this book, I have constantly been helping, advising, and coaching. I would not put anything in here that is not vitally important to everyone's health, whatever your age. Plus, you are part of my Warrior Girls Team, right? You are coachable. You listen to great advice and act upon it. You are smart and have the vision to see the way ahead of you, more than just a few weeks! And you make changes NOW that will set up a better, healthier future. The damage done in the early years of your life can very well catch up with you further down the line.

Your Hormones are potent, but we tend to underrate their influence on our body's functions. They help regulate our weight (more on that shortly), mood, sleep, growth, and a broad range of other tasks that add to our overall health and well-being. We need to look in more detail at the two main hormones controlling menopause: estrogens and progesterone. Decreased levels of these two hormones during menopause can cause many unpleasant symptoms. These hormones are also connected to your menstrual cycle. However, as we become a little older, our levels of these hormones begin to drop. When this happens, our hormonal balance is totally out of sync, which is why you may experience a variety of symptoms during this time, such as mood swings or agitation. Depending upon the severity of your symptoms, your doctor may suggest that you start Hormone Replacement Therapy

(HRT) to help you balance your hormones. HRT effectively replaces the hormones that are low due to approaching menopause. However, that is a choice that every woman must decide for herself, and you should read about the pros and cons of this treatment before you make a final decision.

What you need to understand at this point is that hormones, or a lack thereof, control every aspect of your menopausal experience. This is a natural part of the aging process for a woman and while it can be difficult to understand or deal with, take heart in the fact that it is normal. It is easy to become scared or worried about what is happening to your body when you are starting to notice changes, but remember that you are simply going through a natural process. Recognizing this should help you deal with any anxiety you experience and leave you free to focus on one burning topic.

What Do Hormones Have to Do With Weight Gain?

Unfortunately, the hormonal ups and downs happening during the perimenopausal and menopausal stages mean that you will probably notice a little weight gain. During this time, most women see that they are putting weight on without even trying. You are probably not eating anything different, and you feel that you are not moving any less, but the scales begin to creep up. You will probably notice this particularly around your midriff, the visceral fat I discussed in the introductory section.

There are two things to pay attention to here. Firstly, the confidence issue. There are not many women who are happy to put on weight and simply live with it. It is bound to dent your confidence a little, especially if you notice extra pounds without doing anything to deserve it. Let's be honest. If you have been away on holiday and enjoyed the cakes and wine a little too much, you know that you will have to cut back when you get home. But if you have done nothing to cause this change, it is quite a shock! Weight gain can have an extremely damaging effect on the way you feel about yourself in general. Some women may have had a weight problem in the past, battled to lose it, and felt proud of their efforts (rightly so), only to find that their hormones want to undo their hard work when the menopausal period begins. Quite understandably, this can be upsetting and highly discouraging, affecting not only your confidence but also harming your self-worth.

The second important aspect is that visceral fat can injure your health because it accumulates around the internal organs. This may increase the possibility of developing chronic diseases and severe health conditions such as heart disease, diabetes, stroke, high blood pressure, and liver problems. These are just a few examples of serious health issues, which can damage your quality of life and may even prove to be fatal. Remember that even though menopause can cause you to store unwanted fat around your vital organs, this, of course, usually happens in later life. However, prolonged exposure to refined sugars speeds up the process, chemically altering your body and affecting hormones earlier in our years. We need to do everything we can to reduce these risk factors, to ensure that we all live long and healthy lives. The problem is that this menopausal weight gain can be harder to shift than the weight gain from your younger age. For some reason, you put weight on more easily, yet it will not go away without a fight! It is one of life's rather unpleasant ironies. By understanding why this is happening, you can work out ways to overcome this problem, and I promise you, it can be beaten!

Let's delve a little deeper...

Many studies show that during menopause, the two main female sex hormones, estrogen and progesterone, start fluctuating. Changes in these hormones can lead to developing excess weight around the middle. Your testosterone levels will also decrease during this time in your life, leading to muscle loss as well. Testosterone is the male sex hormone, but women have it too. When you lose muscle, your body will no longer be able to burn fat fast, and you will gain weight easily. This is one of the major reasons I coach and advise women to do strength training. In my 25 years of experience, it is *vital* for ladies to engage in lift exercises! Your muscles will fade naturally as you grow older, but an intelligent lifting program will help slow down this process. And, it doesn't mean you need to live at the gym! Body-weight moves are superb in slowing down muscle loss. Moreover, they actually build muscle! Hormonal imbalance during menopause is known to cause increased appetite and higher food intake. Many women have higher fasting insulin levels and insulin resistance during this period of their lives. This can significantly affect the rate of their metabolism. It causes their metabolism to slow down, and this affects how fast they burn fat. The fact is, the slower you burn fat, the more fat you have. The quicker you burn fat, the less fat you have. A slower metabolism has an adverse effect on the function of the postmenopausal body.

In addition to regulating the menstrual cycle, estrogen is a hormone that is also responsible for managing your weight and ensuring that your metabolism is functioning correctly. It impacts the amount of fat in the body. As you move through perimenopause and into menopause, the slow decline of estrogen (a type called estradiol in particular) can cause your body to store more fat. This results in weight gain and potentially harms bone density, leading to osteoporosis and poor heart health. Hormonal imbalances caused by menopause can affect your sleep quality, and if you are sleep deprived, you are more likely to make poor food choices and reduce the amount of exercise you are doing simply because you are so tired. Lack of sleep will also affect your "hunger" hormones known as leptin and ghrelin. These two hormones are known to influence your hunger level and increase your appetite. As you will learn later in this book, sleep disruption is one of menopause's symptoms, so we have another trigger for weight increase to deal with.

However, please do not despair, because I have plenty of advice on handling this problem and keeping your weight in check. You need to focus your time and attention on becoming healthier, eliminating unhealthy habits, and making good, firm, and positive choices instead. Eating healthy and moving your body more are the two main good habits that can help control your menopausal weight gain, in addition to several other factors. In this book, we have explored many factors and looked at what you need to do to achieve your weight loss goal.

It's so crucial for you to get to know your body. After all, it's the only one you'll ever have! We have many different hormones throughout our bodies, and they are all going to play a huge factor in our mindset. When we talk about hormones, many of us automatically go right into reproductive health, discussing estrogen and testosterone. Some of us are even reminded of those hormonal teenage years when everything seemed so emotional. Maybe you're there now! These are just the stereotypes commonly associated with hormones. As women, you have to recognize they encompass far more than just your sexual health. Hormones play into the way that you sleep, your stress levels, and how you metabolize food. If any one of these hormones is out of whack, it can send everything else in your body into an unhealthy, stormy loop, including your mindset. Our low-carb, low-sugar advice, by its very nature, can help with your mindset because it focuses on hormone regulation. This chapter will cover the significant hormones in women's health" estrogen, cortisol, and insulin, all of which play a direct role in determining how much weight you might be able to lose.

Hormones are special chemical messengers released by various glands and cells in your body. They are carried in your blood and taken to receptors which then activate a signal to make the cells in your body perform a particular function. A good example is the hormone insulin which most people have heard of. This hormone, almost single-handedly, is at the heart of virtually all of the world's chronic health problems. We need to give it tremendous respect and our full attention. It is produced in the pancreas, which is an organ that sits right behind your stomach. When you eat, the digested food is broken down into glucose, the simplest form of sugar that your body has to deal with quickly. Once glucose is released into the bloodstream, your pancreas secretes insulin. Insulin binds with receptors in the cells to take in the glucose to be used as energy. It is important to stress again that the body only needs a small amount of ingested glucose to function perfectly. We DO NOT need every meal to be ¾ full of carbs! The system that takes care of blood sugar levels was not meant to be put under such constant pressure. As we covered earlier in our journey together, girls, our body prefers fat as its primary energy source. Once we have thrown the switch into fat-burning mode, we torch fat from our fat stores, which gives us so much clean burning energy it is unreal! But, it will not burn fat if sugar is present. And, try as we might, we cannot force the body to switch from sugar-burning to fat-burning because it suits us. However, not all is lost. We have a new language, right? And using that language, we can let the body know that it is safe to burn fat because we have nice low blood sugar. It's okay to switch over. Evolution has not caught up with the progress made in making refined goods. And, as we have said before, this can take millions of years! So please do not wait for evolution to change the human body. We need to change our eating habits before chronic illness is too much for our healthcare system to cope with!

Once the glucose moves into your cells, the level in your bloodstream drops, and your pancreas stops producing insulin. If the glucose level drops too much, say you are doing some hard exercise, your pancreas produces the hormone glucagon, which tells the liver to release stored glucose into your bloodstream to keep those hungry little cells fed. Once enough glucose is released and blood sugars are at the level they need to be, the pancreas stops creating glucagon. This feedback system helps keep your body regulated. Too much glucose, and your body produces insulin. Too little glucose, and your body produces glucagon. Similarly, if you are too hot, you will start sweating to cool you down, and if you are too cold, your body makes you shiver to warm up. So, if we are eating too much, our body produces extra insulin to control blood glucose levels, and if we eat less, our body produces less insulin. This is called homeostasis. Homeostasis is essential as it keeps our body regulated. The function of this feedback system is to control blood glucose levels and to regulate blood pressure levels.

Sometimes, however, the stresses of our modern-day life can make these feedback systems go a bit wonky. If the insulin stays high for long periods, the body struggles to deal with it. After using what blood sugar your body can as energy and the liver dealing with what it can, insulin stores the rest as fat.

Simply put, the more highly refined our food is, or how much sugar and fruit we eat, the higher the blood sugar levels, which then forces more and more insulin to be secreted and thus more and more fat to be stored.

By removing the foods that cause blood sugar to spike, we drop the need for excess insulin and burn body fat as fuel.

Not only do we now become leaner, but we also become healthier as excess insulin over a prolonged period is linked to so many chronic illnesses, such as:

- Type 2 diabetes
- High blood pressure
- Skin tags
- PCOS
- Migraines
- Body fat gain
- Liver complaints
- Heart issues
- Eye and feet issues
- And many more

Hormones and Weight Gain

Take, for example, the hormones leptin and ghrelin. Leptin's role is to send signals to your brain to satiate (or tell you when you are full), while the role of ghrelin is to increase your appetite by making you feel hungry. The latest research has shown that chronic sleep deprivation causes ghrelin to increase (causing an increase in appetite). At the same time, the levels of leptin decrease so that it takes longer to signal your brain that you are full, making it all too easy to overeat. Your body cannot replenish its energy through adequate sleep, so it will try to get it through extra food.

Stress can also contribute to an imbalance of hormones and weight gain. When you are stressed, your body produces more of the hunger hormone ghrelin. You also make more of the hormone cortisol, sometimes called the "stress hormone." Cortisol stimulates fats and carbohydrates to be metabolized for quick energy release, which is good in minimal amounts. Stress also stimulates insulin to be released, so that blood sugar levels are maintained, increasing your appetite. These hormonal responses served us well as cave dwellers when we needed the "fight or flight" response to prepare us for fighting off the enemy or fleeing large animals viewing us as lunch. Unfortunately, the stresses of modern-day living can trigger the same "fight or flight" responses and the same hormonal ones too.

What You Can Do To Keep Your Hormones Balanced

If you think that hormones and weight gain are one of your weight loss challenges, here are the two best things you can do. First of all, make sure that you get a good 6-8 hours of sleep a night. Second, try to keep your stress levels to a minimum. If you can't escape from your daily stressors, try to change how you react to them. I found that meditating for 10-15 minutes a day before work worked wonders for me, allowing me to face the day calmer and more focused. Remember, life is a long series of obstacles. Or "stepping stones," as I like to call them. As we approach one of these, take a moment to think of how you intend to deal with it? Stress can be caused by simply not being organized or not having the best plan of attack to get around or over those stepping stones. Take the time to plan each day, just a few minutes each evening before you go to sleep will help tremendously. Also, as we have mentioned before, your subconscious mind will be put at ease knowing what the next day has in store, and you can then totally relax!

> "Life without a plan is like a ship without a rudder or sail. You will eventually end up somewhere, but the 'where' is out of your control. The key is to set a good sail and rudder to end up at the location you planned."

COACH BLADE

Estrogen

Discussions about estrogen usually default to a woman's reproductive system and our various sex organs. In reality, everyone has estrogen, not just female bodies. This critical hormone can affect more than just your reproductive health. It plays a role in skin and bone protection and in helping your body heal bruises and other wounds. When estrogen goes off balance, it can cause different issues in women, depending on your age. Many women struggle with endometriosis or polycystic ovary syndrome. And PCOS is directly linked to chronically elevated insulin levels. Your various estrogen levels can even affect your mood. At the simplest level, you might experience low energy and weight gain because of hormonal imbalances. One concern that women have when starting a low-carb, low-refined-sugar diet is that hormone levels will become unbalanced. Any change in your overall diet can indeed affect your hormonal imbalance. To mitigate this concern, it's essential to understand and know your baseline healthy hormonal levels before you begin cutting carbs and sugar. But remember this, girls, you are not lowering or removing something that the body needs! Sugars and carbs are not an important part of anyone's diet. We would never advise anyone to remove an essential food group required for a long and healthy life! So, removing them will make your body so much better at balancing hormones. It will love you for this one move alone and show that love in looks, feelings, and performance!

To determine if you have a hormonal imbalance, begin by looking at your menstrual cycle. Women with irregular cycles might have issues with their hormonal balance. Whether your periods go on for months at a time, you have painful cramps, or you don't have periods, you should look at your current lifestyle to see if anything there might be the cause. Suppose you have nothing in particular that you can pinpoint as being the cause for this imbalance. In that case, there could be an underlying condition that needs to be treated by a medical professional. Another way that the low-carb, low-refined-sugar diet helps tremendously is by limiting the carbohydrates and sugars that are notorious for throwing hormonal balance awry through fluctuating glucose levels. Also, something as simple as the soap you're using could affect your hormonal balance. It could also be something more medically related, such as an underlying health issue or lifelong condition.

You can also try altering small things in your day-to-day routines to see if it improves any of the symptoms you experience because of a hormonal imbalance. If you're very lethargic or have frequent low moods, ask yourself what might be causing it. Do you lack regular exercise? Is there a life stressor that you're dealing with at the moment? Are there any environmental factors? Once you can pinpoint the possible problem, you can eliminate other factors affecting your hormones other than your nutritional diet. Ensuring your safety and health are the most critical priorities. For women who have severe symptoms of a potential hormonal imbalance, a doctor must first clear this diet since it could cause more serious health issues.

If you have thyroid issues, your estrogen will affect your overall nutrition and digestive system after beginning ketosis. Your body will naturally drop into a ketogenic state as the carbs and sugars are removed. This is perfectly natural and totally the way the body was designed to react. We do not need to measure this. The body will start to burn fat, causing the ketogenic process to start.

You will want to check in with these kinds of hormonal imbalances to ensure that your reproductive health is in normal or acceptable ranges. If you have any hormonal problems while you're in ketosis, there are a few things that you'll want to make sure you're doing correctly. Make certain the food you're eating is nutritional. People often assume that because they are cutting out carbs, they can load up on more dairy or low- to no-carb sugars. You can still indulge every so often, but it needs to be restricted and in small portions. Choosing one diet is no excuse to overeat in another area. Other hormones can also affect your estrogen levels. The next section will discuss cortisol, which is often called the stress hormone. Let's take a look at how it can be affected by a low-carb, low-sugar diet.

Cortisol: The Stress Hormone

Most women know that an estrogen imbalance can affect their mood and how they feel on any given day. Cortisol, the stress hormone, is a crucial factor in mood regulation. When we experience stress, fear, panic, and anxiety, our bodies go through a certain reaction, which releases cortisol through our adrenal glands located just above our kidneys. You're probably quite aware of instances when you've felt stress or fear, but here's an example: You're walking down a path in the forest, when all of a sudden, a snake slithers out of the bushes and stops directly in front of you. Biologically, the first response to something like this is fear, which is also considered stress. This is when cortisol is released, which then initiates your "fight or flight" response. Are you going to confront that snake blocking your path, or will you simply turn around and run the other way?

Regardless of what you choose to do, the biological response to this snake stressor is basically the same: you get that sudden boost of energy, your heart speeds up, your muscles tense, you probably sweat a little to keep you cool and focused. All that buildup in your body is caused by the release of your stress hormone, a.k.a. cortisol. No matter the type of stress we face, work, family, financial, etc., the biological response is the same. It may not be so easily seen or felt, but it's there. More aggressive individuals will likely have the fight response more frequently. Those who are passive and prefer to stay quiet and non-confrontational have a typical flight response. This consistent kind of stress can weigh heavily on your body if you're not managing it.

Of course, stress can be a good thing. For example, when you have a confrontation with a coworker, perhaps it helps improve your relationship, and things get better. Without that initial stress, you might've let issues slide and not cared as much. Stress can be a motivator, and it can remind you of the things that matter most to you. It can also provide clarity and that extra push you need to take risks and try new things. Unfortunately, not everybody is aware of how stress feels to them, so rather than being a helpful biological tool, it's viewed as an inconvenience to be avoided or suppressed. Unmanaged stress can lead to chronic anxiety or depression. When you begin a low-carb, low-sugar plan, there's always a possibility of affecting various hormones, as we discussed in the previous section, but affecting them in a good way! That holds true for cortisol. Losing weight and regulating your overall health can make your body feel better, leaving you energized and happy rather than lethargic and depressed. Also, the stress of a lifestyle change and a chemical change occurring in your body could cause stress. So, in short, a little bit of stress when needed is a good thing. It keeps us sharp and focused. However, high sugar levels will not help our bodies at all. While the body is trying to sort out the high blood sugar, it cannot do anything else. It is THAT important. So reducing sugars will remove so much unwanted stress and give your body a well-earned break!

Insulin Regulation

Insulin is the third hormone that we must pay attention to when starting a low-carb, low-sugar nutrition plan like ours. An insulin imbalance can cause various health conditions. When we hear about insulin, most of us will associate it with diabetes. If you have diabetes, please consult with your physician before going on the low-carb, low-sugar eating plan (I will explain why shortly). If you're not careful with what you eat, you could negatively impact your diabetes, and in severe cases, you could do more damage than good if it's not managed correctly. Even if you do not have diabetes, you're not free from the risk of developing insulin resistance. Let us dive a little deeper into diabetes. Right, my mother has suffered from Type 2 Diabetes (T2D) for over 30 years. In fact, my website and social media pages all spawned from seeing how my mom was suffering, and I wanted to help her and others from around the world as much as possible. Now, stay with me on this statement, girls... If the language of our body is hormones, and at this stage in the book, it is. We are not a big number machine that knows what numbers it has in its stomach. And we also know that blood sugar, if left unchecked, is very dangerous and can be fatal. So, a T2D sufferer has effectively killed off their pancreas by keeping their blood sugar so high, for most of the time, that it simply could not keep up with the demand. "Pancreatic burnout" is what it is known as. Then, because of the constantly high insulin levels in our bloodstream to deal with the high blood sugar, we have so many chronic illnesses as we move throughout life due to those elevated insulin levels. So, my question is this: Why do we treat T2D's by giving MORE insulin? Insulin is the very stuff that has done the damage in the first place! That is like treating an alcoholic with a shot of whisky in the mornings! Sure, they will feel better for a small amount of time, but it will still kill their liver and cause all sorts of health and family problems for years to come, eventually, potentially, becoming fatal!

My little rant is over. Sorry! But listen, girls, if you are or know someone with T2D, they should be staying away from all carbs and sugars. This stuff is lethal for them. HOWEVER! Please note this next part. Go back to your doctor or specialist and chat about adjusting meds/units of insulin to compensate for the lack of high blood sugar. Because if you lower the carbs and sugars, you need to lower your meds, or else you can overshoot and crash your sugars the other way. We want you to use the least amount of insulin you can, beautifully balancing your sugars with diet and not more units of insulin! You stopped your pancreas from working *because* of the high consumption of sugars and refined carbs. Do not keep up the same rubbish diet and expect to inject yourself out of trouble. Your body cannot cope!

That said, let's first discuss what insulin is and how it works.

No matter what it is, your body processes food by breaking it down. The carbohydrates and sugars found in your food are converted into glucose, released throughout your blood, raising your blood sugar levels. As we now know, insulin, made by your pancreas, is the hormone that regulates this entire process. It takes the sugar in your blood and turns it into fat or energy. When the only fats in your body are unhealthy kinds, you risk raising your blood sugar levels too high, which prevents your pancreas from producing the right amount of insulin. The result is that you become insulin resistant.

Whenever the number of free fatty acids throughout your bloodstream is too high, this causes insulin to stop responding properly in the cells of your body. Those who are overweight or obese are at greater risk of developing insulin resistance. But this doesn't mean it can't affect anyone. If your diet is high in fructose, for example, you're more likely to develop insulin resistance. If you're drinking multiple sodas a day, you eat too many sweets, and your diet consists of a bounty of processed carbohydrates, you're certainly at a higher risk of insulin resistance. Even stress can affect this powerful hormone. If you're not exercising regularly, this also puts your body at risk for insulin resistance. You might consider getting tested by your doctor to see if your insulin levels are balanced. You will need to order a special test for this as it is not usually covered in a standard blood test or blood draw. In fact, the body can force sugar levels down by pumping out so much insulin that readings look fine when tested, giving a false positive! Why? Well, the incredibly high insulin needed to make this happen is the real problem here. But it is not tested. So, even though things look well, they're not. The real villain here is the super high insulin levels hiding in the background. But when blood sugar starts to stay high in the tests, only then do you get diagnosed as being a T2D! Despite this, you were already on your way potentially years before as high insulin levels can be tested and detected way before a high sugar reading is seen. So, you could have changed your diet with enough time to not only save your pancreas and health but save so much money wasted on medications you didn't need!

We must begin to regulate the insulin in our bodies. We will talk a little more about insulin shortly as we begin to understand how the body uses food and converts it into energy. As you can see, all of these hormones need to work together to ensure your food is properly digested. If you overlook any of these impor-tant hormones in the course of dieting, it could have several negative side effects on your health. You never want to put your body at risk by being under more stress.

Balancing Hormones

Most important when balancing both estrogen and cortisol levels is making sure you begin your low-carb, low-sugar plan carefully. You'll also want to have a trial and error period to work out any kinks or issues that pop up. If you jump right into the diet expecting to stick to it by the letter, you might be setting yourself up for poor results. It's more important to start slow. Instead of yo-yo dieting for the next three weeks, take one week as a trial to plan and test things out with some flexibility. Gradually change it up to ease your-self into the low-carb, low-sugar plan, and by the third week, it should be easier for you to follow. Of course, everyone will approach this diet differently. Ultimately, it's up to you to figure out what to do that works best for you and your lifestyle. However, because we can now talk to our bodies and know the language of hormones, we can make the better food choices needed to allow the body to stay balanced. Remember that the adverse side effects of estrogen or cortisol imbalances could set you back, discourage you, and cause other health issues that are otherwise avoidable.

Our hormones are sensitive, so anything that might affect them, both good and bad, shouldn't be taken lightly. If one hormone is out of balance, it can also knock all the others out of whack. You can do a few things to make sure that you are harmoniously producing the correct levels of hormones in your body. The first step to take is to ensure you are loading up on probiotics. These are microorganisms that have numerous health benefits. They are essentially good bacteria, and you already have many in your body. These will balance the production of essential hormones needed for over-regulation. Foods high in probiotics are things like Greek yogurt. Be careful when purchasing anything with a flavor since it can be high in sugar and carbohydrates. You'll want to pick whole-fat to get as many of the probiotics needed for overall health as possible.

Fermented foods also offer plenty of great probiotics. Make sure to be cautious of picking foods that are pickled over fermented foods. Fermentation is an actual process in which carbohydrates in food are converted into alcohol. This helps to replenish the good bacteria in your body. Pickling is simply the use of brine as a preservative. Popular fermented foods are things like kombucha and sauerkraut. Jarred pickled foods aren't as good for probiotic use since they have more additives. A ton of food can be fermented, so it's all about personal preference and experimentation. For those that hate anything fermented or dislike dairy and yogurt, you can simply take a probiotic supplement. Any health food store and most grocery stores offer capsules you can take to ensure you are keeping up with your number of healthy bacteria for both mental and physical health.

For hormonal balancing, add a squeeze of lemon or orange to your glass of water or sprinkle over dishes for extra flavor. Citrus fruits are filled with vitamin C, which helps boost the overall production of estrogen within your body. But of course, always be mindful of sugar intake. Stress, sleep, and physical exercise will also affect your hormones, so while you emphasize what you put in your body, remember external factors are important to notice too. Even something like a scented candle can affect your hormones, so note any changes in mood, appetite, and weight loss to ensure your hormones aren't out of balance.

The Impact of Different Hormones

The key players when it comes to weight loss are:

- Cortisol
- Insulin
- Human growth hormone
- Testosterone
- Leptin and ghrelin
- Melatonin and vitamin D

Cortisol

Managing cortisol is probably the most important thing when it comes to fat loss. Chronically elevated cortisol has been strongly linked to visceral body fat, which is the worst kind. Visceral body fat means fat stored around essential organs. Studies are pretty unanimous that visceral body fat is not good for health. It's also the least appealing-looking body fat, and it's got several loving nicknames: beer belly, love handles, and so on.

High cortisol also blocks the secretion of several of the "good guy" hormones. For example, it's borderline impossible to have high testosterone if your cortisol is always high. And cortisol can, of course, wreck your sleep, which will have detrimental effects on all the other hormones. But cortisol is not bad, per se. It's a beneficial hormone. Chronically elevated cortisol is bad. The natural cycle of cortisol goes as follows: it spikes in the morning and then drops. It'll be at its lowest at night. Cortisol will also rapidly spike when you're doing stressful activities such as working out, but then it quickly drops back down. If your cortisol is flowing normally throughout the day, it's a great ally. Only when it's being elevated too often or not allowed to drop back down is when we get into trouble.

Only elevate cortisol when you need the energy, such as when working out and doing very intensive work. Try to keep cortisol down as much as you can throughout the day.

Cortisol elevation is essentially the same as stress. There's no need to bring cortisol up actively. It'll go up whenever you're doing anything that elevates your heart rate or engages you intensely. That's all fine and useful. Remember all the tips and tricks to managing stress from the previous chapter? Be mindful of those.

Outside of your stressful activities, try to stay calm as much as possible during the day, and if something startles you, try to bring yourself back down to baseline as fast as possible. Don't embrace stress. Try to relieve yourself from it.

Insulin

Insulin is the primary driver of fat storage. To over-simplify a bit: your fat cells wouldn't take in fat without insulin sending the signal. So it's almost impossible to gain body fat if your insulin is low. This is the key thing to understand. But insulin also drives muscle growth and other good things in the body. It's not bad. It's just potent. As with cortisol, you want to elevate insulin at the right times and keep it low at other times. Fortunately, this is quite easy with insulin. Carbs and protein are the only things that significantly elevate it. When do you want high insulin? When you want the body to grow. After exercising, your body is primed to use insulin in muscle growth. If you haven't exercised in a while and spike insulin, your body will want to store the additional energy as fat.

Testosterone

Testosterone builds strength, be it in the body or the mind. And remember, it doesn't matter if you're a man or a woman. You want your levels to be in the healthy range. Since testosterone strongly contributes to muscle growth, it's also beneficial when it comes to weight loss. Studies show that testosterone treatments help obese and overweight people to lose body fat and not lean muscle when they are calorie-deprived. That's the result you'll want as well. Remember that the goal is better body composition, not just weight loss. Testosterone is similar to human growth hormone because high-intensity exercise and sleep are the most important factors to consider. But managing your cortisol is a close third. Chronically elevated cortisol will blunt your testosterone production like nothing else. These two are strongly inversely correlated.

Leptin and Ghrelin

As we discussed earlier, leptin is a satiety hormone, and ghrelin is a hunger hormone. There's really no need to get super scientific with these two. If your goal is weight loss, it's pretty clear you don't want to feel hungry all the time. The easiest way to manage hunger is to eat fewer carbohydrates. Carbs evoke a strong feeling of hunger (through ghrelin), whereas proteins and fats make you feel satisfied (through leptin). That's not to say that carbs don't have any effect on leptin or that fats and protein won't elevate ghrelin, but the effects in both cases are more negligible. Avoid Processed carbs, embrace fats and protein.

What happens to these hormones when you combine lots of fats, protein, and carbs in a single meal? When a meal has large quantities of all three, the body can still only deal with the glucose generated from the carbs. In short, the body will store the fat you eat in that meal because the carbs trigger the insulin loop. The key is to remove the processed carbs from the meal so that the body consumes fat for fuel instead of storing it.

It's also worth saying a couple of words about artificial sweeteners. People assume that artificial sweeteners such as those found in Diet Coke are benign for weight loss because they don't have any calories. This is true in the strict calories in, calories out model, but as we've already covered, that model does not work well in real life. Artificial sweeteners "trick" the body into thinking it's eating something sweet, and so the body prepares itself for increased blood sugar. When blood sugar rises, the body releases insulin as a response. This feedback loop will ultimately make you feel full via leptin, and you'll stop eating. But because artificial sweeteners don't have sugar in them, your blood sugar doesn't rise. Instead, you just elevated your insulin for no reason, and there's no leptin secretion to make you feel full. So not only are you craving more sweet foods because of a lack of leptin, but you're also unnecessarily spiking your insulin and setting the stage for fat storage. Artificial sweeteners are also linked to all kinds of unfortunate consequences, such as gut bacteria dysregulation. The bottom line is clear: you're making your fat-burning lifestyle more difficult by ingesting artificial sweeteners.

Beyond diet, there is one other thing that is very important for proper leptin and ghrelin functioning. You guessed it: sleep, of course. When you don't get enough sleep, you end up with too little leptin in your body, which makes your brain think you don't have enough energy for your needs. So your brain tells you you're hungry, even though you don't actually need food at that time, and it takes steps to store the calories you eat as fat so you'll have enough energy the next time you need it. The decrease in leptin brought on by sleep deprivation can result in a constant feeling of hunger.

Melatonin and Vitamin D

No surprises here. You want to sleep when it's nighttime and be awake and outside when it's daytime. A healthy circadian rhythm is vital to all hormone functions. Look back to the chapter on sleep for tips on getting a good night's rest and make sure to get enough sun exposure during the day to raise your vitamin D levels. Or, if it's wintertime, supplement with vitamin D.

Chapter Summary

Goodness me! Now that was some deep stuff, right? But now, can we all see that numbers play no part in our health or body fat percentage? It is ridiculous to think otherwise!

Key Points -

- Insulin controls body fat. Control your insulin, and you can control your body fat levels.
- Lack of sleep and stress can crush all aspects of fitness and health. Learn to control them.
- "Middle age spread" has nothing to do with overeating as we get older. We are simply becoming more insulin resistant. But do not worry, this can and will be helped by following our guidelines in this book.

FINAL WORDS

WEIGHT LOSS MIGHT NOT BE the most straight-forward task to complete, but luckily, you know by now that achieving it is only the final stage. Many of the benefits you're looking for actually start to manifest much sooner, and you now know enough to help yourself get there. You haven't been given a strict diet to follow like a machine, but you have been given enough tools and grounding for you to make healthier adjustments to your diet. You can proudly say that you better understand what makes certain foods good for you and what makes them nothing but filler. As humans, we tend to focus on our physical bodies because we experience the world in a physical sense. Our ego wants us to look good and feel healthy, and that is a good thing. Healthy and fit people live longer, and the longer you live, the more time you have in this lifetime to realize your potential, fulfill your mission, and accomplish your "why."

When you are unhappy with your weight or feel bad about your appearance, it sucks up a lot of emotional energy and mental focus. When you get healthy and lose weight, you will find you can now focus more of your time and energy on something besides worrying about your health or how you look in the mirror. Decide now what you want your mission to be, and any challenges you face with change will be easier. Losing weight and getting healthy is undoubtedly beneficial, but your mission in life is about more than just you. I hope you found the mental health aspects of this journey interesting and entertaining as well. Meaningful weight loss isn't all about its physicality, and long-term health improvements require a mindset that supports and cherishes self-care.

Going forward, don't be afraid to seek out further knowledge if needed, and don't forget that not all of it has to be directly related to weight loss either. Any technique or activity that genuinely improves your health is worth learning about, regardless of whether or not it changes how much force gravity exerts on you. You are worth caring about, one way or the other, but only you can be there for yourself 100% of the time. Don't let the mistakes of your past go to waste, and be your own champion. Take a holistic approach to your health.

Ultimately, the take-home message from me and this book is this:

> *"For ultimate metabolic health, lower body fat and tons of energy... It's no secret. It is simply keeping the refined carbs and sugar low in your diet, add in intermittent fasting and some regular exercise, and you will have it all, FOR LIFE!"*

COACH BLADE

For additional tips, support, and to take an active role in your health and wellbeing, please don't hesitate to reach out!

Discover more on my website:

https://iscfitness.co.uk/

And get involved by joining our community on Facebook:

https://www.facebook.com/ISCFitnessUK/

I'll see you there!

Image Credit: Shutterstock.com

Printed in Great Britain
by Amazon

80159721R00120